3 4028 10711 4085
HARRIS COUNTY PUBLIC LIBRARY

W9-CNB-422

When used properly, plants provide a wealth of healing powers. Adaptogens (plant extracts that help the body adapt to stress) and herbs are some of the most potent sources of such energy and immunity—plus they have a host of additional health benefits. Cookbook author and blogger Jennifer McGruther of Nourished Kitchen expertly guides readers through the properties of herbal energetics and how to gain the most from these dynamic sources. Jennifer explains each function and application, and how to extract their benefits into tinctures, infused oils, teas and tisanes, vinegars, and more. And while store-bought adaptogenic powders and elixirs from popular retailers may be a hefty investment, Jennifer's creations cost only a few dollars to make at home.

Vibrant Botanicals provides more than 70 recipes for helping you feel your best when using herbal infusions. You'll discover how cacao and licorice naturally awaken the body and can be incorporated into granolas, beverages, and breakfasts to jump-start your day. Garlic, astragalus, reishi, and more are showcased in homemade broth and fire cider to help build immunity; while passionflower, ashwagandha, and chamomile are mixed into creamy milk blends and teas to ensure peaceful sleep.

Whether you are looking to fortify digestion, lift your spirits, or just enjoy a good night's rest, *Vibrant Botanicals* provides the natural solution, through nourishing and herbal-rich recipes.

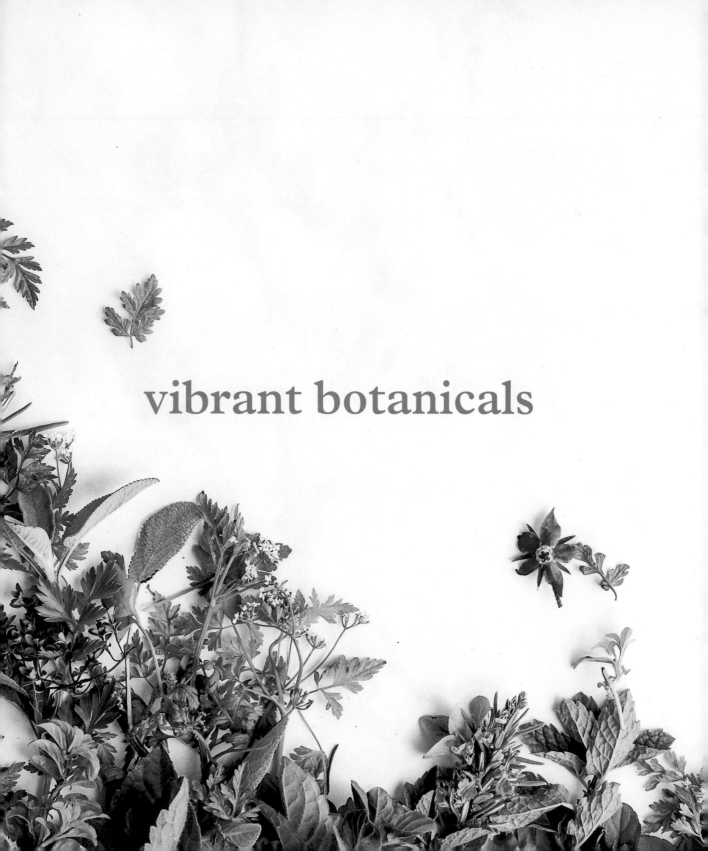

vibrant botanicals

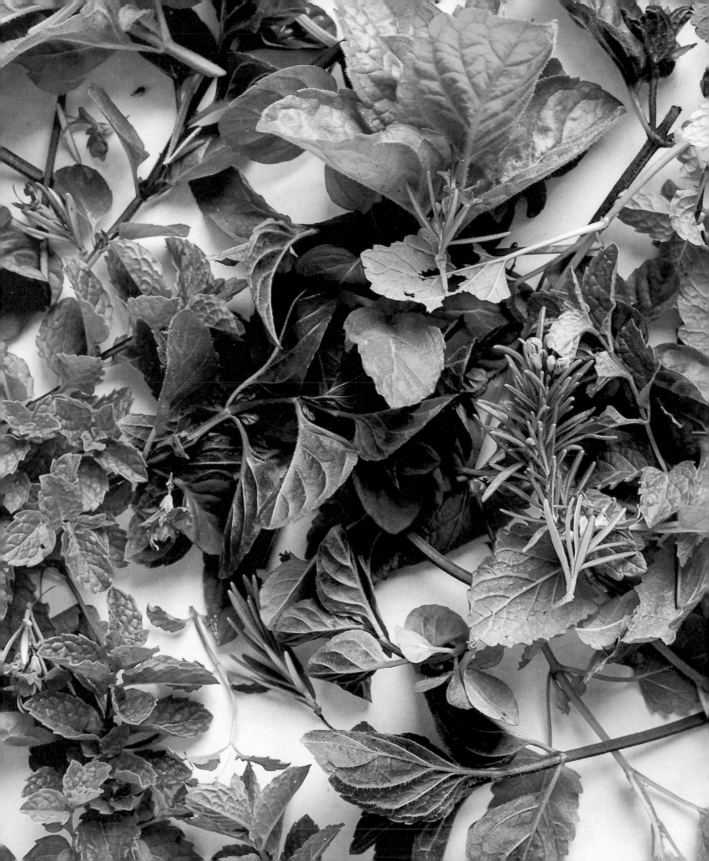

vibrant
botanicals

transformational recipes using
adaptogens & other healing herbs

Jennifer McGruther

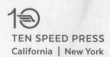

TEN SPEED PRESS
California | New York

contents

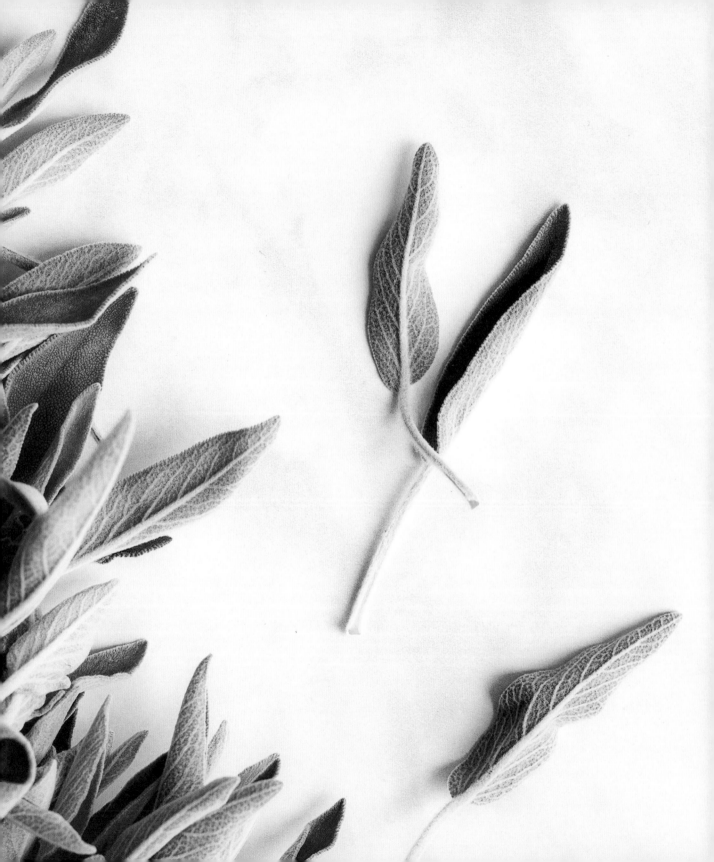

introduction

Growing up, I had a fascination with plants. I sipped sweet honeysuckles freshly plucked from the vine, nibbled on violets and dandelions, and sampled the herbal tisanes an elderly neighbor brewed. Each herb resonated for me on an energetic level. They spoke to my hunger for nature, connection, and deep nutrition.

Later, I began growing my own herbs: I tended terra-cotta pots filled with odd mints, speckled sages, lemon thyme, purple basil, and rose geraniums. Feverfew and chamomile grew like tiny daisies in the garden alongside angelica, valerian, anise hyssop, lavender, and unruly bushes of rosemary. By the time my oldest son turned four, he could recognize a few dozen plants by their leaves alone. In spring, we'd head to the woods to gather nettles, wild rose, and self-heal. Then in fall, we'd pick rosehips and cinnamon-capped bolete mushrooms.

Herbs are essential in our kitchen, and they satisfy a genuine hunger for connection. More than just satisfying flavor, herbs hold a profound and transformational power, tapping into your body's innate healing wisdom. Moving with intention and grace, you can harness these properties to support immunity, ease a headache, boost your energy on drowsy mornings, or help you relax on restless evenings. When used as an adjunct to a nutrient-dense diet, adequate sleep, and gentle movement, herbs can also enact even more powerful transformations: lifting the mood, boosting memory, and blunting the effects of stress.

While herbs aren't cure-alls, they are powerful tools that bring life to your meals while drawing on ancient healing traditions. Most important, they empower you to get in touch with your intuition, take the lead in your health, and reclaim lost culinary traditions in which food and medicine were synonymous.

As you work through this book, remember that every herb you toss into your stockpot or scatter over a platter of freshly sliced fruit brings a gentle botanical medicine to your dishes. The botanical profiles throughout these pages will help acquaint you with the herbs you can use in the kitchen, what they do for the body, and how they work energetically.

It's a powerful feeling to toss a palmful of wild and unruly herbs into your sauté pan with the knowledge that you're nourishing yourself and the people you love in a deeply connected way. Choose the herb-forward recipes with mindfulness and strategy. Sip on a mug of Immunity Broth (page 108) when you feel under the weather. Start your day with a bowlful of granola spiked with cacao and stress-busting adaptogens (page 28), or make a batch of Iced Sencha tea (page 59) when you need to concentrate.

Lastly, keep flavor at the forefront of your mind because good flavor is good medicine, too.

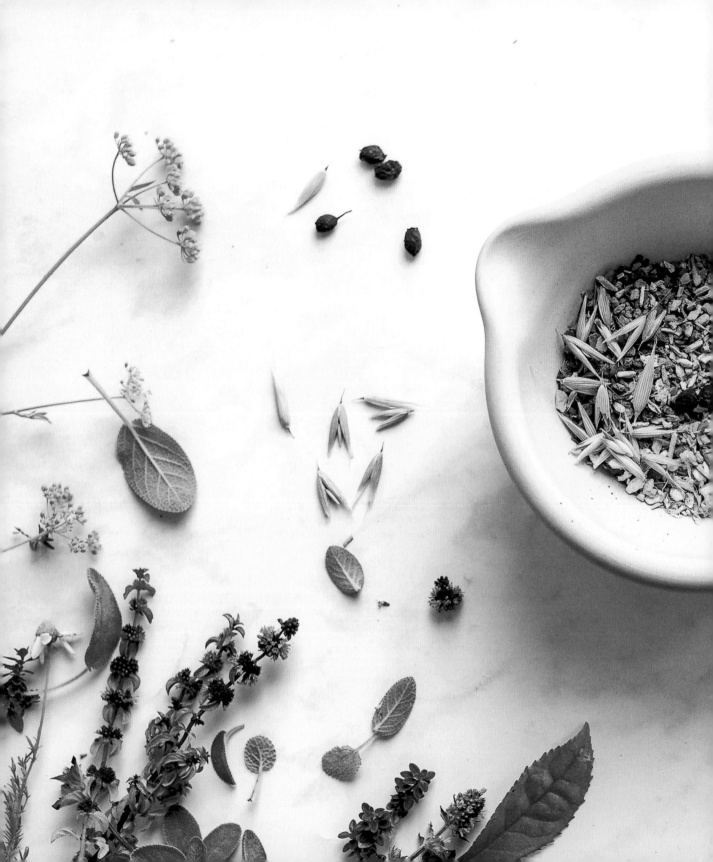

CHAPTER 1

kitchen medicine

When you think of herbs, you might think of little leafy plants, potent with flavor, such as basil and thyme. Spices, by contrast, you know as the tough plant parts such as gingerroot or peppercorns with their heady aromas. There's another way to think of herbs, too—one that's rooted in folk medicine. In this way, an herb is any edible plant that you value for its medicinal effects, aromatic qualities, or flavor. From this perspective, spices like turmeric and cardamom and even flavor-forward vegetables like garlic and onion are herbs just as much as parsley and chervil.

Honoring the healing potential of botanicals in addition to their flavor empowers you to cook with intention and purpose. When you add a spoonful of grated ginger or chopped fresh garlic to a pan, you infuse your meal with rich flavor. Yet, beyond flavor, you bring a distinct and ancient medicine to your meals, too. Cooking with herbs draws upon primal traditions and a time when both food and medicine were inextricably linked.

Herbs give life to your food. Their pronounced flavors and penetrating aromas bring a distinct character to the foods you make with them. Cinnamon brings warmth to meals, and mint cools the palate. The same plant compounds that give herbs their distinctive taste also give them their benefits. What makes cacao bitter also gives your body energy. The aromatic, citrusy notes in cardamom come from the same compounds that also pacify systemic inflammation and support digestion.

These gentle but potent medicines often work best with time and consistency. In the kitchen, you can harness this power and cook to both satisfy hunger and nourish yourself more deeply and intentionally. A spiced tea made with immune-supportive herbs warms you on winter days and also fortifies your immune system against cold and flu season, while a salad made from bitter dandelion greens provides both nourishment and digestive support.

As you cook with herbs, explore your senses. It's a sensual experience that allows you to develop a sense of self-trust and, more importantly, cultivate self-care that is otherwise missing in a world that continually demands more of you.

Lean on your senses and your intuition. Explore what resonates with you and what pleases you on an energetic level. Take the time to enjoy the feeling of sage leaves, soft as a lamb's ear, as you pluck them from the stem. Crush rosemary between your fingertips so that you can take in its aroma. Toss fresh mint into your water and feel how it cools and refreshes your body. As you work with herbs, you'll come to know their personalities and their energies, putting both to work in your kitchen.

herbal energetics

Each herb has a vital energy. Herbalists categorize these energies in pairs of opposites, and they include warming/cooling, drying/ moistening, stimulating/relaxing. Broadly, these energetic binaries describe how herbs affect your body. Herbs have more than one energy; for example, mint is both cooling and drying while thyme is warming and stimulating. Where herbs rest on an energetic spectrum helps you understand how and when to use them.

You already tap into these energies, though you may not know it consciously. If you've ever sipped ice-cold mint tea on a hot summer afternoon, you'll recognize the way it refreshes you, providing coolness and relief. You might crave a warm curry, perfumed with cinnamon, ginger, and chiles on a cold winter night. You tune into your body's need for stimulating energy when you begin each morning with coffee.

These energies also work best in balance with your body's energy, the energy of other herbs, and the weather or seasons. Consider how, during the coldest months, traditional winter dishes feature warming herbs, such as pumpkin pie spiked with ginger and cloves or mulled cider touched with cinnamon. By contrast, in the summer months, you might crave icy mint teas or cooling cucumber salads served with chopped fresh parsley.

warming herbs

warming herbs

basil, black pepper, cardamom (see page 135), cayenne, cinnamon, coriander, fenugreek, garlic (see page 92), ginger (see page 128), licorice (see page 31), marjoram, rosemary (see page 65), thyme (see page 99)

Warming herbs stimulate circulation and digestion and raise the pulse. Chiles taste hot and fiery, and they can also irritate your skin when you chop them. Cinnamon brings warmth to wintertime pastries. This class of herbs is useful when the weather turns gloomy. They can be particularly helpful in combating a cold. Many herbs that we associate with cooking are warming herbs because they support digestion and are a natural match for food.

cooling herbs

cooling herbs

borage, cilantro, elder (see page 117), hibiscus (see page 112), lavender (see page 207), lemon balm (see page 168), lemongrass (see page 176), mint (see page 146), rose (see page 197), stinging nettle (see page 43)

Cooling herbs mitigate inflammation, reduce irritation, and settle nervous tension. Serving an herbal infusion made with hibiscus and mint is refreshing on a hot day, while a hot cup of lavender and lemon balm tea can settle the nerves. They're useful in hot weather when your body needs relief from the heat and can be helpful when you feel generally inflamed, too.

moistening herbs

Moistening herbs encourage moisture in your skin and in your tissues. So, if you have dry skin or a hacking dry cough, these gentle and soothing herbs bring energetic balance. For people prone to fluid retention or congestion, moistening herbs may be less helpful than drying herbs.

moistening herbs

borage, chamomile (see page 217), fenugreek, licorice (see page 31), savory

stimulating herbs

Stimulating herbs can boost your energy levels, increase circulation, and excite the nerves. Herbs such as black pepper and ginger can stimulate good digestion, while others, such as cacao and tea, stimulate the nervous system, which results in increased energy and focus. These herbs also amplify the energy of other herbs and bring harmony to blends. Herbs that stimulate the nervous system, such as licorice or coffee, are best consumed early in the day.

stimulating herbs

basil, black pepper, cacao (see page 27), cardamom (see page 135), cinnamon, ginger (see page 128), licorice (see page 31), oregano, thyme (see page 99), turmeric (see page 82)

relaxing herbs

Instead of stimulating the body, these herbs have calming effects and release pent-up tension. With their quiet and pacifying energy, they work best in the evening. You might serve them in a dessert such as Blueberry Apple Compote with Chamomile Whipped Cream (page 221) or toss a blend of lemon balm and lavender together for an evening tea. Some herbs can be both stimulating and relaxing, working along two or more different pathways in the body. For example, chamomile can relax the nervous system while also stimulating digestion.

relaxing herbs

chamomile (see page 217), lavender (see page 207), lemon balm (see page 168), mint (see page 146), rose (see page 197)

drying herbs

Drying herbs help clear excessive moisture, such as when you're struggling with phlegm from an upper respiratory infection. They also encourage sweating, which is helpful when you have a fever. Many herbs in this category have an astringent or tannic quality, such as sage.

drying herbs

cayenne, elder (see page 117), fennel (see page 141), lemon balm (see page 168), mint (see page 146), rosemary (see page 65), sage (see page 72), stinging nettle (see page 43), thyme (see page 99)

the flavor of herbs

We experience herbs through our senses of taste and smell. Taste is the perception you experience when certain compounds light upon your tongue, and smell is the perception you experience when you inhale those compounds. In addition to taste and aroma, herbs will relay a physical sensation in your mouth. An astringent herb will give your mouth a dry feeling, just like a tannic wine. Chiles may make your mouth feel warm and hot, while mint may cool it. Flavor combines all three—taste, aroma, and sensation—and excellent flavor combines them in a way that pleases your senses and satisfies your palate.

Flavor has beneficial effects on your body. Just experiencing the taste of bitterness or acidity can stimulate and support digestion. Tasting sweetness can provide comfort and satisfaction, while craving salt often signifies a need for minerals. Like an herb's energy, these flavors balance one another.

sweetness

Sweetness is what you experience when you taste both complex and simple sugars. It's a satisfying flavor and nourishing, too. Sweet foods and herbs build strength. A platterful of roasted carrots, which turn sweet and begin to caramelize in the oven, taste delicious and help satisfy and strengthen your body. Sweetness also speaks to an energetic need for comfort. Maybe you crave sweets when you feel anxious or stressed.

The standard American diet emphasizes hyper-sweet foods as well as salty foods. Processed foods are heavily sweetened to increase palatability, and, culturally, sweet foods tend to overshadow bitter or sour foods. The need for sweetness speaks to our culture's collective need for comfort, connection, and quick energy. While sweetness, as a flavor, is desirable, purposeful, and even beneficial, it's easy to consume out of balance. Enjoy concentrated sweeteners, such as honey and sugar, in smaller amounts and favor more nutritive sweet foods such as root vegetables, whole grains, pulses, nuts, or fresh fruits as staples of your diet. Incorporate sweet herbs, such as vanilla or cinnamon, to satisfy that need for comfort.

saltiness

Saltiness is a nourishing and grounding flavor, signifying the presence of minerals in your food. Sodium tastes salty and is the key mineral in table salt, but potassium tastes salty, too. In natural foods, these salt-forward minerals occur in concert with other trace minerals. Unrefined sea and rock salts contain mostly sodium chloride, with trace amounts of calcium, iodine, lithium, and other minerals. A serving of leafy greens contains some naturally occurring sodium and potassium as well as calcium, iron, and magnesium, while a handful of pumpkin seeds contains a small amount of sodium in the company of abundant calcium, phosphorus, and zinc. Sometimes, consistent cravings for salty foods might indicate a need for more mineral-rich foods overall. These minerals nourish your body and are responsible for a wide range of essential bodily functions. They support nerve function, bone health, muscle contraction and relaxation, fluid balance, as well as the formation of various hormones.

sweet herbs

cinnamon, cloves, fenugreek, cooked garlic (see page 92), lemon balm (see page 168), mint (see page 146), rose (see page 197), vanilla

salty herbs

caraway, celery seeds, chives, garlic (see page 92), parsley, stinging nettle (see page 43)

Salt enhances flavors and makes your food taste good. But ingesting too much table salt in the absence of other mineral-rich foods leads to imbalance. If you find yourself craving salt, try using unrefined sea salt with its full complement of trace minerals and add other mineral-rich foods to your diet, such as sea vegetables and leafy greens.

bitterness

Bitterness is the flavor you experience when you taste compounds in plants called alkaloids as well as certain amino acids, which are related to proteins. As a flavor, bitterness excites the digestive process. If you've ever bitten into the pithy rind of a lemon and felt a buzzing sensation in your jaw, you'll understand the physiological effects of bitterness. Bitterness kick-starts digestion, stimulating the release of saliva and digestive enzymes that help you make use of the nutrients in your food more effectively. Bitter foods can also support your body's natural detoxification pathways through the liver and gallbladder, while promoting better blood sugar balance.

For many people, bitterness tastes unpalatable and unpleasant, but it can bring balance to other flavors. Endive, chicory, and other leafy greens taste mildly bitter and are easy to incorporate into your meals. Many culinary herbs have a bitter flavor, too.

bitter herbs

chamomile (see page 217), citrus peel, cumin, dandelion (see page 154), lavender (see page 207), oregano, rose (see page 197), rosemary (see page 65)

sourness

Sourness is the sensation you experience when you taste something acidic. It's the bright flavor of lemons, blackberries, vinegar, and yogurt. As with bitterness, eating sour foods and herbs can stimulate your appetite and kick-start the digestive process. Sourness balances heavier foods and is a great companion for supporting your body's ability to better digest dietary fats. Acidic foods also help your body better use the minerals in your foods, and they make a good companion for leafy greens and other mineral-rich foods.

sour herbs

hibiscus (see page 112), lemon balm (see page 168), lemongrass (see page 176), rose (see page 197)

pungency

Pungency is a catch-all term for any intensely aromatic or hot and spicy herb. Pungent herbs complement sweet and salty flavors. Like bitterness, pungency can spur digestion, and these herbs typically have a warming energy because of the fiery sensation they create in your mouth. Ginger, chiles, raw garlic, and black pepper all taste pungently hot. It's not all about heat, though. In addition to hot and spicy herbs, this class of botanicals also includes deeply aromatic plants. Herbs whose aroma is sharp, with a powerful flavor, are also pungent herbs. Neither rose nor saffron taste hot, but their aromas are striking, deep, and strong.

pungent herbs

basil, black pepper, cayenne, cilantro, cinnamon, cloves, coriander, cumin, garlic (see page 92), ginger (see page 128), lemongrass (see page 176), rose (see page 197), rosemary (see page 65), sage (see page 72)

These herbs stimulate the senses and excite the palate. Too much can overwhelm your senses, leading to unpleasant physical sensations or indigestion. If you've ever eaten too many chiles or too much garlic, you know the feeling.

astringency

astringent herbs

cacao (see page 27), coffee, oregano, rose (see page 197), sage (see page 72), tea (see page 57), thyme (see page 99)

Astringent foods can leave your mouth feeling dry. It's the parched sensation you experience when you taste red wine, coffee, pomegranate juice, or dark chocolate. Like sourness and bitterness, astringency stimulates digestion. More important, these foods also support your body's detoxification pathways.

Astringent foods and herbs act to tone your tissues, calm inflammation, and support your body on a cellular level. The anti-inflammatory effect of astringent foods comes from their plentiful array of polyphenols, micronutrients you find in many plants. These compounds help reduce cellular stress caused by free radicals, and researchers associate them with better systemic health. They're particularly useful in their support of better blood sugar balance and heart and cognitive health. Cruciferous vegetables, beans and lentils, and red berries tend to taste astringent.

how herbs work within the body

While reflecting on an herb's energy and flavor will help you understand how it broadly works on the body, it's also worth exploring the specific functions, or actions, of each herb. Just as an herb may taste of one or more flavors, it will also have more than one action. The botanical compounds responsible for herbal actions vary. As composites of nature, herbs work in a multitude of ways. Chamomile, with its soft-petaled flowers and apple-like flavor, both supports digestion and calms the nervous system. Sage supports mental clarity and also soothes a sore throat. Saffron, with its high antioxidant content, promotes cognitive health while also lessening anxiety.

Unlike drugs, which are synthesized, concentrated, and standardized to contain a specific chemical, at a specific concentration and for a specific purpose, herbs are wildly unruly. Their botanical compounds will vary depending on climate, growing conditions and methods, and even the season in which it was picked. That's because herbs, at their heart, are nature-based medicine. Nature is both wild and unpredictable.

finding the right herb

Discovering herbs that you both enjoy and that also fulfill your targeted health needs is a process of both knowledge and intuition. Learn about how herbs work while also reflecting on which herbs resonate with you both energetically and with respect to how they taste. Give yourself permission to explore what you enjoy and discover what makes you feel good, on an energetic and physical level. As you move through the kitchen, tap into your intuition and what feels right to you.

Does the herb resonate with you? Sometimes, an herb will somehow feel right. Try a new herb for a few days, incorporating it into your meals to see how you feel. You might sip lemon balm tea in the evenings to see if it lifts your mood, or try incorporating licorice into your morning routine to see if it improves your energy levels. You can toss fresh herbs into salads or use them to garnish your meals, and dried herbs make delicious spice rubs. Sipping an herbal infusion is another simple way to learn whether or not an herb resonates with you.

Does it do what you want it to do? Look for herbs whose actions, or how they work within the body, align with your goals and emphasize these herbs in your cooking. If you need more energy in the morning, look at the recipes for starting your day (see page 23), or if you find yourself plagued by digestive troubles, try some of the tea and bitters recipes in chapter 5, "Recipes to Support Digestion." Each chapter in this book provides guidance on choosing herbs with strategy and intention so that they work for your needs.

Do you enjoy its flavor? Herbs bring flavor to your meals. Sometimes the fiery bite of ginger or the salty mineral-like qualities of stinging nettle are precisely what you need to bring a recipe to life. Herbs that taste potent or even harsh may resonate with you right away, or you may find that it takes time to learn to love them. Either way, when cooking with herbs, always let pleasure and good flavor take the lead.

Is it sustainably and ethically produced? Overharvesting threatens many medicinal herbs, such as American ginseng and chaga mushroom, while exploitative labor practices pose a problem in the production of other plants, such as cacao and tea. Choose sustainably grown, responsibly gathered from the wild, and ethically farmed options to minimize any negative impact your choices have on people and the planet.

You can grow many of your own medicinal and culinary herbs in small spaces or in containers, or try sourcing them locally so that you can feel assured of their quality and the way they've been produced. The Resources section (page 226) lists many sources for herbs from companies that take organic agriculture, ethical wildcrafting, and labor rights seriously.

using herbs safely

Herbs hold a potent medicine within their roots, leaves, flowers, and seeds, and most herbs are safe for most people to consume. Small amounts can enliven the foods you make with beauty, radiant flavor, and medicinal compounds, and when you take larger doses over time, they exact more powerful transformation. If you take herbs therapeutically, that is, intending to treat a condition or alleviate a symptom, make sure to do so under the guidance of an appropriately qualified health care provider.

Be careful when using herbs in the following circumstances:

You're pregnant or trying to conceive. Traditionally, herbalists used botanical medicine to support fertility and reproductive health; however, some herbs, such as rosemary and angelica, may threaten pregnancy, especially when you take large doses, as in supplements and tinctures. If you're pregnant, it's generally safe to consume herbs in the small amounts you'd normally use when you cook, but always talk with your health care provider before using herbs medicinally or in large amounts.

Further, some herbs will cross through the placenta, which means that the herbs you take may affect your baby. Tea, coffee, cacao, and other plants that contain caffeine are widely considered acceptable in small amounts, but they may affect your baby if you consume them in large amounts or too frequently. Fortunately, there are many you can take safely during pregnancy such as dandelion (see page 154), stinging nettle (see page 43), mint (see page 146), and chamomile (see page 217). Always work with a qualified health care provider who can help you decide which, if any, herbs are appropriate for you.

You're breastfeeding. Just as the active compounds in some herbs can pass through the placenta to a developing baby, they can also pass through breast milk to a nursing infant. Many herbs are well suited to both you and your nursing baby, but others may create cause for concern. Certain herbs, such as garlic, may upset a young baby's stomach, while others, such as tea or cacao, may overstimulate the baby. Often research is simply lacking, and there's too little information to make a safe recommendation.

If you're nursing, work with a qualified practitioner to pinpoint appropriate herbs to use, and inform both your health care provider and your child's pediatrician if you're using any herbs therapeutically.

You're giving herbs to a child. Culinary doses of herbs are safe for children, as they are for most other people. Remember, though, that children's bodies are small and sensitive. An herb that's benign or even beneficial for an adult may overwhelm a child. Gentle herbs with long histories of use, such as mint (see page 146), stinging nettle (see page 43), and fennel (see page 141), are best for children. Use them only in fractions of adult doses. Further, make sure to work with your child's health care provider and always let them know any herbs you've given your children.

You take medication. Certain herbs, especially in large doses, may interact with medications. Some herbs may increase the efficacy of the medicine you take, while other herbs may dull its effects. Both ginger and turmeric can slow blood clotting, so for people who have bleeding disorders or who take blood thinners such as warfarin, it's best to avoid these herbs. Similarly, fenugreek supports blood sugar balance, and because of these effects it may cause hypoglycemia in people who take medication for diabetes. So always let your health care provider know which herbs you take and talk with them before adding new herbs to your routine.

You have a health condition. Herbs are beautiful companions to life-style changes, and they can help enact meaningful transformations in the way you live and feel in your body. Yet, they're also an adjunct to medical care, and not a substitute for it. So, if you have a health condition, always work with a qualified health care provider to determine an appropriate treatment plan.

You have allergies, intolerances, or sensitivities. Since herbs are members of botanical families, you might find that you react to different plants within the same family. So, an herb that might otherwise support wellness in another person may cause you distress. For example, if you find yourself sniffling and sneezing when ragweed blooms, consider avoiding other members of the daisy family (Asteraceae) such as echinacea or chamomile. If nightshades such as tomatoes and egg-plant give you an upset stomach or itchy skin, you'd do well to avoid medicinal herbs in that family, such as ashwagandha, regardless of their benefits. Lastly, if you try an herb and it doesn't sit well with you, causing you stomach distress, anxiety, headache, or other symptoms, avoid it in the future. Other herbs are likely a better fit for you on a bio-individual basis.

growing, buying, and storing herbs

The easiest way to have access to fresh herbs throughout the year is to grow them yourself. Growing your own is also both affordable and pleasant, and it's something you can do even in small spaces. Most herbs do just as well in containers as they do in garden beds, so a few potted plants on your patio or windowsill can give you ready access to fresh herbs. Of course, if you haven't the time, energy, or space to grow your own, buy fresh herbs at a local market and high-quality dried herbs at well-stocked herb shops and online (see Resources, page 226).

A reputable herb shop will be able to tell you how and where the herbs they sell were grown. Most shops stock organic herbs, meaning the plants were grown without synthetic agricultural inputs. Brick-and-mortar shops may also specialize in herbs from local growers who practice organic agriculture, but may lack official certification due to the small scale of production. You'll also find wild-crafted herbs in many well-stocked shops. Instead of coming from farms, these herbs are gathered from wild sources. While overharvesting poses a risk to certain wild plants, ethical wild-crafting focuses on sustainable harvesting techniques that help ensure the viability of wild plant sources for future generations.

Buying fresh herbs. Look for lively herbs with perky leaves and plump stems. If you can, snap off a leaf and roll it between your fingers. Does it release a sharp and clear aroma? If so, it will convey a beautiful flavor to the meals you make with it. In the kitchen, store herbs with tender leaves, such as mint and parsley, in a small jar filled with water. Cover them with a loose-fitting plastic bag and keep them in the refrigerator, changing the water daily. For herbs with woody stems, such as thyme and rosemary, wrap them in a slightly damp cloth to prevent them from drying out and place them in an airtight container. Fresh herbs will keep their vibrancy for about 1 week in the refrigerator.

Buying whole dried herbs. Whole herbs are dried and minimally processed, and they include star anise pods, cardamom pods, vanilla beans, cinnamon sticks, and other herbs that are as close to their original form as possible. Whole herbs will retain their volatile oils better than ground herbs, and you can grind them fresh in a spice grinder or with a mortar and pestle just before using them for better flavor. You can also toss whole herbs into infusions and broths. Store whole herbs in tightly sealed containers away from direct light and heat. Whole herbs are shelf-stable, but try to use them within about 3 years before their flavors and medicinal compounds wane.

Buying cut and sifted herbs. Cut and sifted herbs are dried herbs that have been coarsely chopped and then sifted to remove the dust and small bits of debris that result from processing. They are perfect for slipping into infusions and what you'll use most when you make these recipes. Look for herbs with strong aroma and good color. Faded herbs may have been improperly stored or may have lost some of their medicinal benefit. Store cut and sifted dried herbs in tightly sealed containers away from heat and direct light. Properly stored, they should keep about 1 year.

Powdered herbs. Shops sell many herbs as finely ground powders for convenience. You'll find small glass bottles filled with golden-orange turmeric powder, sweetly scented ground cinnamon, and scarlet-colored paprika. Powdered herbs are more likely to be adulterated than whole or cut and sifted herbs, so buy them from a reputable source. Store ground herbs in tightly sealed jars in a cool spot in your kitchen away from direct light. Like cut and sifted dried herbs, they'll keep about 1 year.

how to use herbs

Both culinary and medicinal herbs are diverse. You can use them in many different ways in your kitchen, releasing both their flavors and healing energy into the foods you cook. For some, it's as easy as swirling a bit of olive oil in a hot pan and tossing in the herb, while others need more exacting methods to extract their benefits.

fresh and raw

Herbs taste delicious and vibrant when you use them fresh. For basil, mint, cilantro and other leafy and aromatic herbs, add them at the very end of cooking or scatter them over your dish right before serving. Add chopped fresh herbs to salads or to bring a little brightness to dessert. You can also make sauces and pestos (by blending herbs with oil, nuts, or seeds) to swirl on top of eggs in the morning or add interest to a plate of roasted vegetables at dinnertime.

powders, dust, and salts

Freshly ground herbs give your foods delicious, robust flavor owing to the release of essential oils that can dissipate quickly after grinding. Toss whole herbs and spices into a spice grinder or grind them by hand with a mortar and pestle. Toasting them in a hot pan just before you grind them releases more volatile oils, and that translates to rich and penetrating flavor.

Spices, such as seeds, barks, and roots, work well for making powders and dusts. Dredge meat and fish in freshly made herb powders before grilling or roasting or try sprinkling a pinch of herb dust over roasted vegetables.

decoctions, tisanes, and infusions

When you steep herbs in hot water, you prepare an herbal infusion. Sipping warming tisanes soothes and comforts the body, while drinking cold infusions can be refreshing. Infusions are the most popular way to enjoy many herbs because they taste pleasant and are easy to make. You can make them with fresh herbs in season and dried herbs throughout the year. Due to the high water content of fresh herbs, you'll need to use roughly three times the volume of fresh herbs as you would dried for the same effects.

Different herbs, however, require different approaches to preparing the most beneficial and nutrient-dense infusion. Hardy, tough herbs release their compounds best when boiled in water and then allowed to steep, while delicate, leafy herbs are best simply steeped in hot water rather than boiled. Further, if you intend to make the most nutrient-dense and medicinal infusion, you'll likely need to steep those herbs for several hours or even overnight for the greatest benefit. Infusions lose their vibrancy after about 3 days in the refrigerator. While most are pleasant served cold over ice, if the weather's cold, you can also warm them up just before serving them.

decoctions

Decoctions are concentrated infusions that you make by boiling herbs and then allowing them to steep in hot water. Boiling helps hardy herbs, such as licorice root or star anise, release their compounds more efficiently, especially when you begin by tossing the herbs in cold water and allowing it to come to a boil gradually.

recipes that use this technique

chicory and dandelion latte (page 38) and spiced astragalus tea (page 122)

basic decoction

2 tablespoons hardy, tough herbs such as roots, bark, or seeds

2 cups cold water

Add herbs to a saucepan, cover with cold water, and then bring to a boil over high heat. Immediately turn down the heat to low, allowing the herbs to simmer for about 20 minutes or until they color the water and release a deep aroma. Strain the decoction through a fine-mesh sieve into a jar or, for a stronger brew, let the herbs continue to steep for several hours until the liquid cools to room temperature before straining. Decoctions will keep for about 3 days in the refrigerator.

tisanes

To make a tisane, briefly steep fresh or dried herbs in hot water, just long enough to release a delicate flavor. You might also know tisanes by the more common term *herbal tea*. Tea, in a technical sense, refers specifically to the tea plant (*Camellia sinensis*) and the drink you make with it. To differentiate between true tea and delicate herbal infusions, I've used the term *tisane* in this book. Tisanes taste pleasantly mild, with a soothing and refreshing energy. Use delicate plant parts such as leaves and flowers when you make tisanes. Because the herbs spend less time in hot water than they do in decoctions or overnight infusions, tisanes are less potent.

basic tisane

─────

2 tablespoons cut and sifted dried herbs (or 6 tablespoons fresh herbs)

2 cups boiling water

Spoon the herbs into a heatproof jar or into a tea strainer set into a large mug. Cover the herbs with boiling water, allowing them to steep 5 minutes. Strain and enjoy right away, or transfer it to the refrigerator until cold. Tisanes will keep for up to 3 days in the refrigerator, but tend to lose their potency quickly.

nourishing infusions

Unlike tisanes, which steep just long enough to release their aromatics, nourishing infusions steep at least several hours and often overnight. While decoctions taste robust and tisanes delicate, nourishing infusions have a concentrated flavor that signals deep nutrition. These infusions tend to have a richer nutrient profile than tisanes alone. Like tisanes, delicate plant parts work well for making nourishing infusions.

basic infusion

─────

¼ cup cut and sifted dried herbs

2 cups boiling water

Scoop the herbs into a heatproof jar. Pour the water over the herbs, then let them steep for at least 4 and up to 12 hours. Strain and enjoy right away or transfer it to the refrigerator for up to 3 days. Serve cold or warm on the stove before serving.

oils, vinegars, and ghee

You probably use oil or vinegar every day in your cooking. Maybe you swirl a few tablespoons of olive oil in the skillet in the morning to fry eggs or dress a salad with olive oil and red wine vinegar for dinner. When you infuse these fundamental ingredients with herbs, you can bring bold flavor to your meals in a new way. It takes very little effort but plenty of patience to make herb-infused oils and vinegars.

Herb-infused ghee is finished in less than an hour, while other infusions take a little more time and patience.

herbal ghee

Ghee is clarified butter (in which the milk solids have been removed), used in traditional Indian cookery. Ghee, like olive oil and other cooking fats, preserves the flavor and benefits of herbs beautifully. Cardamom and fennel work nicely in ghee, as do garlic and rosemary.

recipes that use this technique

bedtime tisane (page 206), energizing morning elixir (page 37), iced sencha with spearmint and ginkgo (page 59), midnight flower tisane (page 214)

recipes that use this technique

nettle mint infusion (page 51), tulsi and lemon balm lunar infusion (page 165)

spiced ghee (page 135),
three-herb ghee (page 64)

basic herbal ghee

1 cup unsalted butter

2 tablespoons whole herbs or cut and sifted dried herbs

Melt butter in a wide skillet set over low heat until it froths and foams. Then toss in the herbs, allowing them to slowly release their flavor into the golden-rich butter. The creamy milk solids will begin to separate from the rich butterfat, sinking to the bottom. When the milk solids begin to brown, it's time to strain the ghee into a clean jar. After straining the ghee through a cheesecloth or butter muslin, discard the solids. Use it as you would butter. Homemade herbal ghee will keep for about 3 months at room temperature and up to 1 year in the refrigerator.

herbal oils

Always use dried herbs when making herb-infused oils. Fresh herbs can pose a food safety risk since their low acidity and high water content can leave your oil vulnerable to botulism. Making herb-infused oils is an exercise in patience and relaxed intuition, and you can use them in place of olive oil in cooking, on salads, or drizzled over a plate of roasted vegetables or meat.

rosemary and sage oil
(page 67)

basic herbal oil

½ cup cut and sifted dried herbs

1 cup oil, preferably extra-virgin olive oil

Fill a pint-sized jar with herbs, and then cover them with the oil, allowing about 1 inch of headspace. Seal the jar, label it, and tuck it in a cupboard away from direct light and heat for 1 month. After a month, strain the oil and remove the herbs. Store the oil at room temperature, away from direct light and heat for up to 1 year.

herbal vinegar

Vinegar's potent acidity extracts plant compounds easily and with little coaxing. As a result, herb vinegars are flavor-forward. Garlic and chiles give vinegar a startling punch, while the softer notes of tulsi or chamomile bring an aromatic quality to the vinegar. Apple cider vinegar is affordable and easy to find, but you can also use wine vinegars, if you prefer their flavor. Herb-infused vinegars can enliven a dish of earthy beans or roasted vegetables with a hit of much-needed sourness. Herbal vinegars are also the foundation for another popular herbal remedy: oxymel. Oxymels are herbal drinking vinegars to which honey has been added for palatability.

basic herbal vinegar

▄▄▄▄▄▄▄▄▄

⅔ cup fresh or dried herbs

1 cup vinegar

Place the herbs inside a pint-sized glass jar, and then pour in the vinegar. Seal the jar with a plastic or nonreactive lid and then transfer it to a cupboard away from direct light and heat. Let it rest about a month, shaking the jar daily to agitate the herbs. Then strain the vinegar through a fine-mesh sieve into a bottle, discarding the solids. It'll keep indefinitely, but I like to use it within about 1 year.

herbal honey

Honey's sweetness comforts and soothes. Many herbs work well in honey, but floral and aromatic herbs such as lavender, rose, coriander, and cardamom work best. These herbs, with their striking aromatic compounds, complement honey's floral undertones. Sweetness softens bitter notes and is a pleasant way to take herbal medicines whether that's a spoonful of rose-infused honey in your morning yogurt or a spoonful of honey, lemon, and ground cinnamon during the cold and flu season.

basic herbal honey

▄▄▄▄▄▄▄▄▄

½ cup fresh or dried herbs

1 cup honey

Spoon the herbs into a pint-sized jar. Then fill the jar with honey, allowing about 1 inch of headspace. Using a chopstick, stir the herbs into the honey so that they're well coated and suspended rather than floating on the surface. After about 1 month, strain the honey and discard the herbs. Herbal honey keeps in the cupboard indefinitely, but I usually use it within the year, preparing a new batch when the herbs come into their season again. Use herbal honey to sweeten tisanes or desserts.

tinctures and bitters

Tinctures are alcohol-based herbal remedies made the same way as herbal oils and vinegars. Since you take only a small amount, ½ teaspoon to 1 teaspoon at a time, they're often a more palatable way to consume (and enjoy the health benefits of) bitter or less pleasant-tasting herbs. Bitters, including those used in cocktails and aperitifs, are a type of tincture made with bitter-tasting herbs. Herbalists

recipes that use this technique

fire cider with rosemary and sage (page 97), raspberry tulsi vinegar (page 167), garlic and thyme oxymel (page 100), strawberry shrub with schisandra and chamomile (page 183)

recipes that use this technique

honey-fermented garlic with bird's eye chile (page 94), vanilla rose petal honey (page 198)

traditionally use bitters to support digestion before meals, while other herbal tinctures convey a variety of benefits depending on the herb you use. Motherwort tinctures ease worry and support mood, while tinctures made from hops and chamomile can help you sleep. You can use both herbal tinctures and bitters in your own cocktails or stir them into sparkling water or nonalcoholic elixirs if you prefer.

Herbalists begin by macerating single herbs in high-proof alcohol such as 100-proof vodka, then they strain the herbs and blend the tinctures together, as a perfumer might blend essential oils into a perfume. For beginners, I recommend the simpler approach below.

basic herbal tincture

½ cup fresh or dried herbs

1 cup 100-proof alcohol, such as vodka

Add the herbs to a pint-sized jar Next, cover the herbs with alcohol, allowing about 1 inch of headspace. Let the herbs steep for about 1 month away from light and heat and shake the jar daily. Strain out the herbs, preserving the tincture, and store it in the cupboard for up to 2 years.

recipes that use this technique

bedtime bitters (page 222), citrus ginger bitters (page 132), echinacea and astragalus tincture (page 121), motherwort tincture (page 187)

equipment

When you work with herbs, you'll need to keep a few extra tools in your kitchen. While you likely have almost everything you need already, take the time to look over this list. Keeping the right equipment on hand makes cooking a little bit easier and a lot less frustrating.

Fine-mesh sieves: Most recipes call for straining herbs, and a fine-mesh sieve works well because it catches even the smallest bits of leaf or stem. You can find them in a variety of sizes; it's nice to have a large sieve for straining herbal broths, while small strainers, just large enough to fit snugly in the mouth of a jar, work well for infusions, oils, vinegars, and tinctures.

Glass jars: Glass jars in a variety of sizes ranging from a pint for tinctures to 2-quart jars for broths and infusions make preparing herbal remedies easier. Use jars both to store herbs and to store the remedies you make from them.

Vials with eye droppers: Store tinctures and bitters in small glass vials fitted with eye droppers so they're easier to use.

preventing corrosion
in metal lids

Vinegar and other acidic ingredients corrode metal, especially with prolonged exposure. So when you make herbal vinegars or tinctures, use plastic or other nonmetal lids. If you only have access to metal lids, line the lip of the jar with a square of wax paper and then seal the jar as you normally would. The wax paper forms a barrier between the vinegar and the metal lid, helping to prevent corrosion.

Spice grinder: They're small and affordable and grind dried herbs efficiently in very little time. Freshly ground herbs taste stronger and more intense than store-bought preground spices. A spice grinder also makes it easy to blend various herbs together for rubs, powders, and dusts.

Mortar and pestle: Like a spice grinder, a mortar and pestle allow you to grind herbs. While less efficient than an electric spice grinder, using a mortar and pestle allows you to grind herbs by hand—a rhythmic and meditative task that can help you get in touch with the herbs you use in your kitchen.

Kitchen scale: You can measure herbs with measuring cups and spoons, but kitchen scales allow you to measure ingredients by weight, providing more accuracy and consistency in your cooking.

Funnels: Having both wide- and narrow-mouthed funnels makes it easier to transfer your remedies into jars and vials with minimal spillage. I recommend using stainless steel funnels, which you can find in well-stocked kitchen supply stores and online.

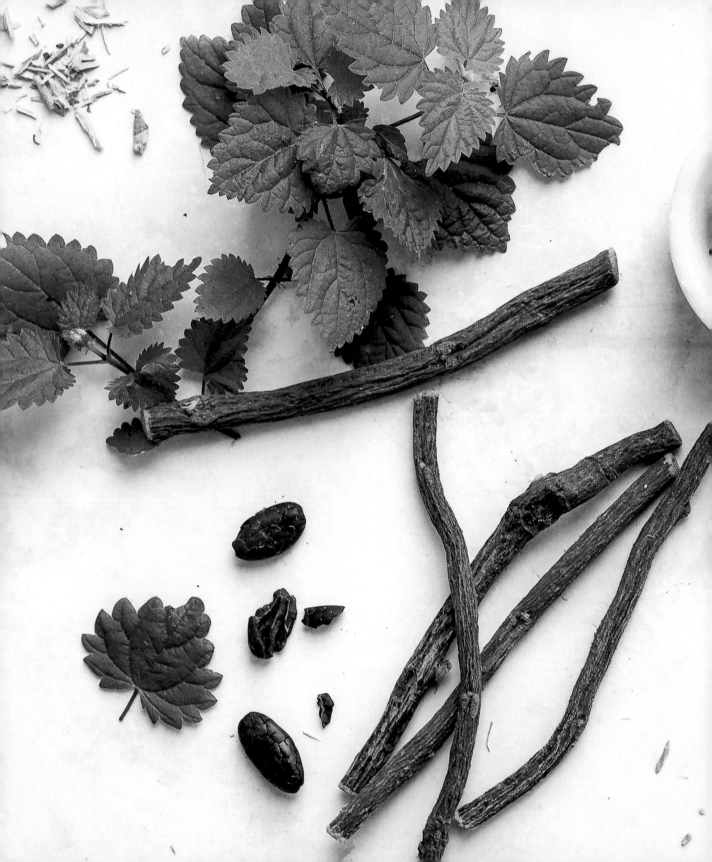

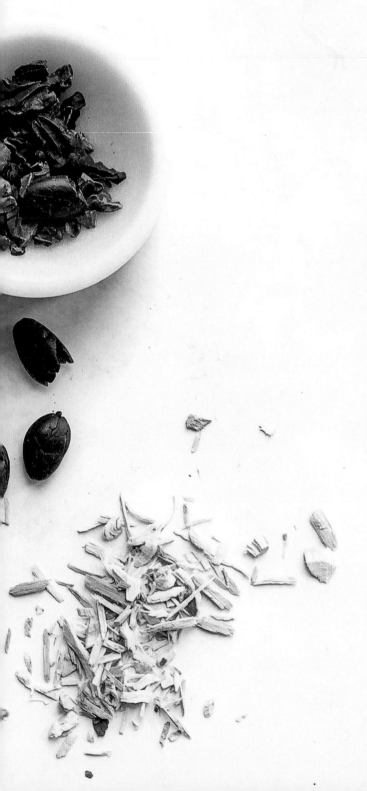

CHAPTER 2

recipes to
start your day

Morning is a time for renewal. It's a time to breathe deeply, prepare for the day ahead, and nourish yourself in a way that makes you feel alive. The daily morning rush, however, may leave you more brutalized than energized. Still exhausted from yesterday's unending workload and responsibilities, you rouse yourself from bed hardly ready to start the day. While you deserve to wake with clarity and stamina, it feels like a constant game of catch-up that you can never win.

Medicinal plants can't give you an extra hour in the morning, but they can set the foundation for an easier day. Whether you toss herbs into your breakfast or brew them into an infusion, you tap into a sense of nourishment and connection. This simple element of self-care can transform your morning and your day. I lean on three distinct types of herbs in the morning: those that nourish, those that build resilience against stress, and those that increase energy in a sustained way.

herbs for the morning

Nutrient-dense herbs: Nutritive herbs have plentiful vitamins and minerals that build and nourish your body. Stinging nettle (see page 43), red raspberry leaf, alfalfa, and oatstraw are popular, and they're rich in vitamins C and K as well as silica, magnesium, phosphorus, and other minerals, respectively.

Herbs that ease stress: Adaptogens help your body respond to and build resilience against stress. They support your adrenal, hypothalamus, and pituitary glands. These glands form your body's stress-response system. Some adaptogens, such as licorice (see page 31) and eleuthero (see page 35), have a secondary, stimulating effect. These stimulating adaptogens work well in the morning. Others, such as ashwagandha (see page 192), can quiet the nervous system, making them ideal any time of day.

Energy boosters: Stimulating nervines are herbs that boost your energy. These invigorating herbs work well in the morning to energize your body and mind. Some plants, such as coffee, are more stimulating than others. Others, such as tea (see page 57) and cacao (see page 27), have a milder effect. If you use them daily, you might find you crave them or that their energizing effects seem to diminish over time. When used too often or in large amounts, they can also increase jitteriness or anxiety. If you've ever had too much coffee, you know the feeling. I like to use these herbs from time to time rather than daily.

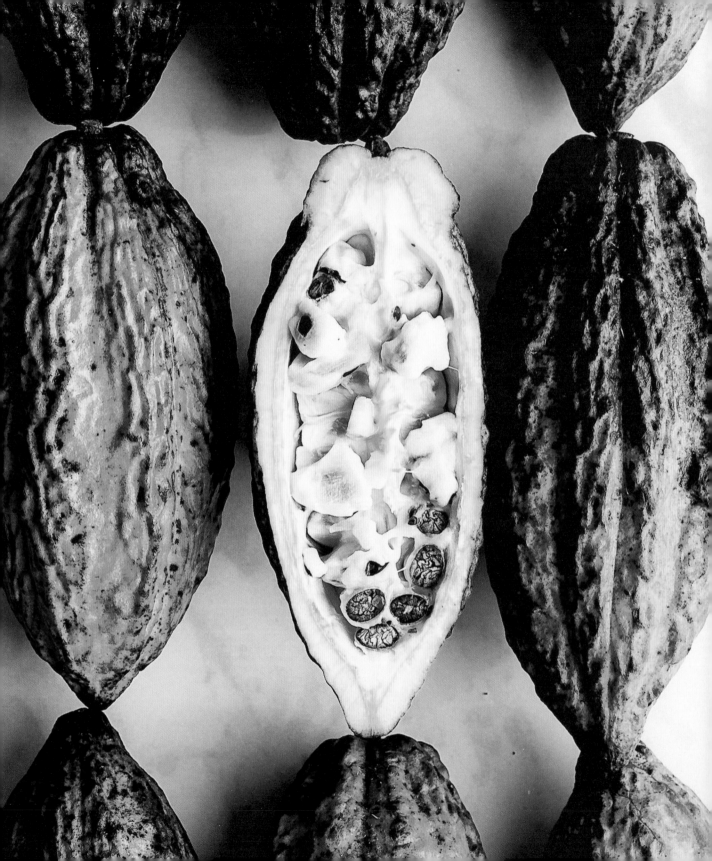

cacao

(theobroma cacao)

The cacao tree is an evergreen in the mallow family, which also gives us hibiscus (see page 112). Its hard pods range in color from vivid yellow to earthy red, and they hold large, fatty seeds. Producers process the seeds to make raw cacao nibs and powder, cocoa powder, cocoa butter, and chocolate. These foods are indulgent, nutritive, and medicinal all at once.

Cocoa and cacao powders taste similar, faintly bitter with a chocolatey aroma. The primary difference between the two is that beans for cocoa powder are roasted, while beans for cacao powder are not. This means that cocoa powder typically has a richer, toastier aroma. From a nutritional perspective, cacao and cocoa powder are a good source of magnesium and copper.

Cocoa butter is rich in saturated fat and contains vitamins E and K.

While the cacao plant is a nutritive food, it also contains medicinal properties. It's exceptionally high in flavonols, which are potent antioxidants that help support cellular and cardiovascular health. These compounds increase blood flow to the brain and improve brain function while also reducing systemic inflammation.

Cacao also contains theobromine, a bitter alkaloid related to caffeine. Like caffeine, theobromine stimulates the nervous system and dilates the blood vessels. Its ability to dilate the blood vessels makes chocolate a good choice when you feel a headache coming on; however, it may trigger migraines in sensitive people. Because chocolate stimulates the nervous system, it can also energize your body when you need it, making it an excellent choice to start the day or when you need a mental boost in energy.

Take care in choosing your cacao products, too. Cacao is cultivated throughout the world, including Latin America, Southeast Asia, and Africa. More than 70 percent of the world's cacao is grown in West Africa, where the demand for cheap chocolate has sped the deforestation and mass destruction of rain forests. Further, the chocolate industry depends heavily on the labor of trafficked and enslaved children. Choose certified fair-trade cacao products when possible.

Using it in the kitchen: Cooks typically pair cacao with sugar and milk, which dulls its beneficial effects. Simmer the nibs in hot water and then strain the cacao-infused liquid to make a drink similar to coffee. You can also use cacao nibs as a topping, as you would nuts and seeds.

dark chocolate granola with raspberries

MAKES ABOUT 8 SERVINGS

1 cup sprouted rolled oats

½ cup chopped raw walnuts

¼ cup sliced almonds

¼ cup chopped raw hazelnuts

¼ cup cacao nibs

⅓ cup maple syrup

¼ cup cocoa butter

½ teaspoon fine sea salt

¼ cup cacao powder

1½ teaspoons eleuthero powder

½ teaspoon rhodiola powder

1 cup freeze-dried raspberries

Bittersweet with notes of maple, this simple, energy-boosting granola is an excellent way to start the day. You can prepare it in advance, over the weekend, and toss it into jars to pair with yogurt for an easy grab-and-go breakfast for the week ahead.

Cacao provides a mild, stimulating energy balanced by two adaptogens: eleuthero (page 35) and rhodiola (page 39). These two herbs work in concert with one another to help fortify your body against stressors, increase stamina and mental clarity, and give you a boost of early-morning energy.

One of the charms of this recipe is its versatility. While cocoa butter gives the granola a rich, chocolatey flavor, you can use coconut oil in a pinch. I like to use sprouted rolled oats for their sweetness and because they're easier to digest and plentiful in bioavailable minerals, but you can use old-fashioned rolled oats instead, and you can always swap the eleuthero and rhodiola powders for more cacao if you prefer.

Preheat the oven to 250°F.

In a large mixing bowl, toss the oats, walnuts, almonds, hazelnuts, and cacao nibs. Stir them together until well mixed.

In a small saucepan over medium-low heat, warm the maple syrup and cocoa butter. When the cocoa butter melts, whisk in the sea salt and the cacao, eleuthero, and rhodiola powders. Pour the cocoa butter mixture over the dry ingredients and then stir well to coat.

Spoon the granola mix onto a baking sheet and bake for about 40 minutes, stirring once or twice to promote even cooking.

Remove the baking sheet from the oven and let the granola cool to room temperature. Break up any large pieces and then toss in the raspberries.

Transfer the granola to an airtight container where it can store for up to 1 month in your cupboard.

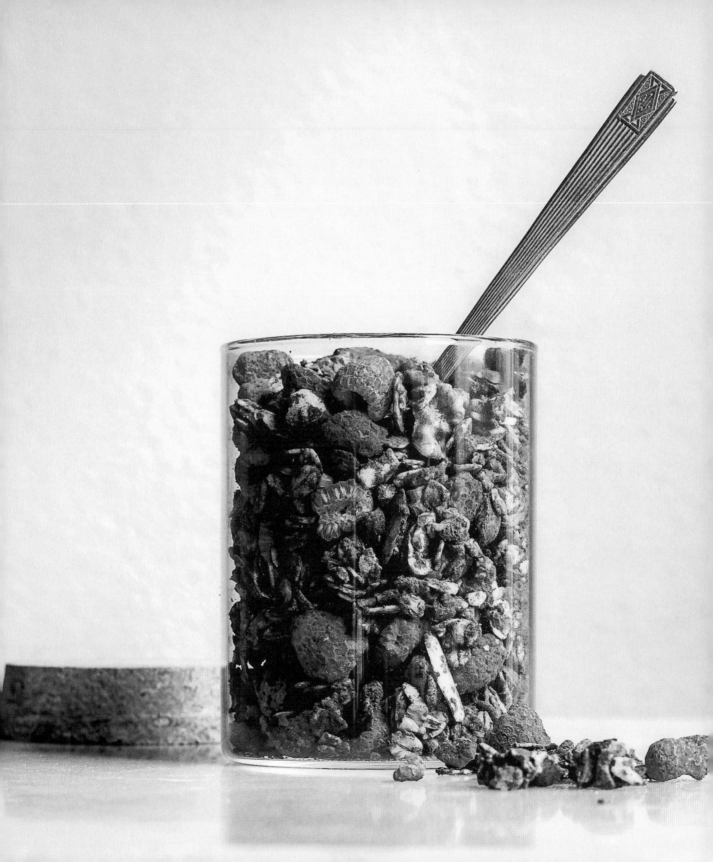

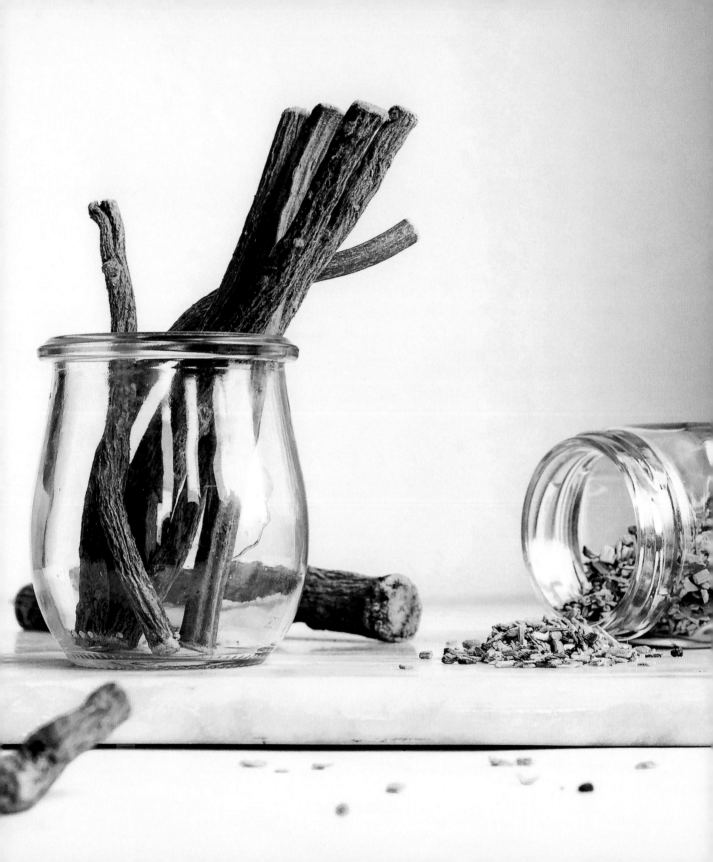

licorice
(glycyrrhiza glabra)

Licorice grows about 3 feet tall in spindly stems, saddled on either side by matching oblong green leaves. It blooms in the summertime with pale purple flowers, and while they're lovely to look at, it's not the flowers you want. Instead, it's the long, woody roots that hold the plant's magic and medicine.

The roots, when dried, look like small logs or the kindling for an elfin fire. While you can chew on the cleaned roots as they are, you'll most often find them dried and coarsely chopped or ground into a fine powder. Unlike black licorice candy, real licorice tastes pleasantly sweet with no hint of anise. Its sweet flavor makes it generally well-liked and a great companion for bitter-tasting herbs. It harmonizes herbal blends, softening the harsh flavor of other herbs and helping them work together synergistically.

Like other adaptogenic herbs, licorice buffers your body against chronic stress. Beyond that action, it supports hormonal and metabolic health, which are so keenly interlinked.

Because licorice supports the adrenal glands and has a gently stimulating quality, it can give you a boost of energy. So, take it in the morning before noon and avoid using it close to bedtime.

Using it in the kitchen: Use powdered licorice root to sweeten drinks or add it to homemade truffles and date bars. You can make a decoction from licorice root by tossing it in a pot, covering it with cold water, and bringing it to a boil. When the water begins to boil, turn the heat to low and let it simmer for about 20 minutes before straining. Avoid prolonged use of licorice, which may be linked to electrolyte imbalances.

cherries poached in licorice and black tea

MAKES 4 SERVINGS

2½ cups cold water

1 tablespoon cut and sifted dried licorice root

2 teaspoon cacao nibs, plus more for serving

1 vanilla bean, split (optional)

1 star anise pod

1 tablespoon black tea, such as Darjeeling

1¼ pounds fresh or frozen sweet cherries, pitted

½ cup honey

Yogurt for serving

Yogurt and fruit make an excellent breakfast: simple, fast, and satisfying without feeling heavy. If you tire of fresh fruit, try poaching it instead. Herbal infusions make a delicious poaching liquid, especially when coupled with honey or another natural sweetener. In this recipe, black tea and cacao give poached cherries a deep flavor that's brightened by the aromatic notes of star anise. The effect is both robust and delicate.

Hardy herbs such as roots, stems, and seeds take time to release their flavor and benefits, and tender, fragile fruits can't stand up to this increase in time and heat. To solve that riddle, prepare your poaching liquid in advance, which allows you to simmer the herbs the length of time they need to yield their aroma and goodness. Then, once the herbs are spent and you've strained the infusion, you can swirl in the sweetener and begin poaching the fruit until they're cooked through but still firm enough to give you a good bite.

In a medium saucepan over medium-high heat, combine the water, licorice, cacao nibs, vanilla bean (if using), and star anise, bring to a boil, and then immediately turn down the heat to medium-low. Simmer, uncovered, for about 15 minutes.

Turn off the heat and toss in the black tea. Cover and let the herbs steep for an additional 5 minutes.

Strain the infusion through a fine-mesh sieve into a 1-quart jar, discarding the solids. Wipe the saucepan clean.

Return the liquid to the saucepan and bring it to a boil over medium-high heat. Immediately turn down the heat to medium-low and then stir in the cherries and honey. Simmer, uncovered, for about 5 minutes, until the cherries are warmed through but not soft. Turn off the heat and let it cool to room temperature.

Serve over yogurt, sprinkled with additional cacao nibs.

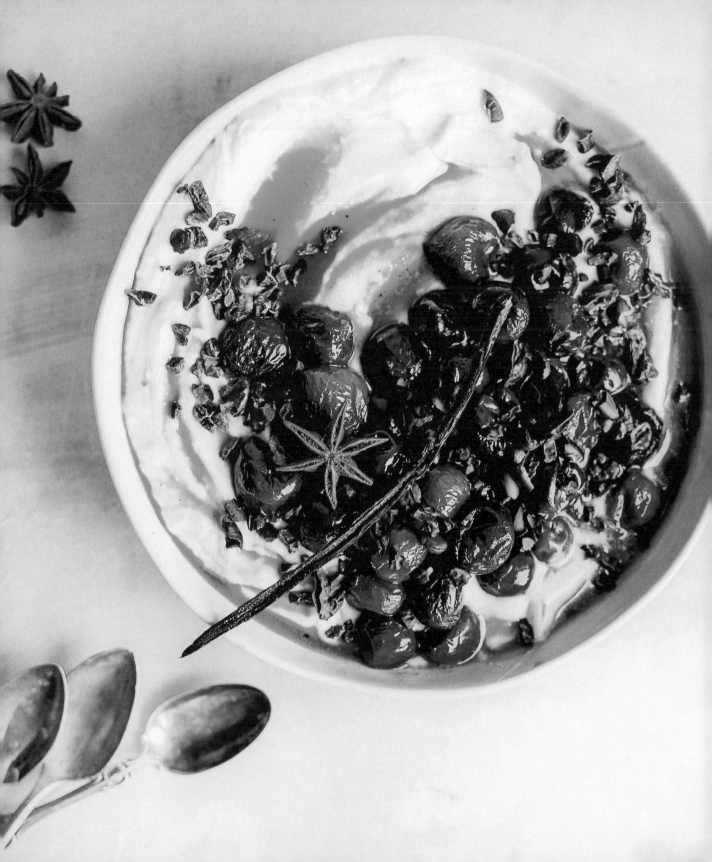

flaked rye porridge with sautéed apricots

MAKES 4 SERVINGS

porridge

2 cups flaked rye

1 teaspoon apple cider vinegar

1 teaspoon fine sea salt

4 cups apple juice

apricots

1 tablespoon Spiced Ghee
(page 136) or unsalted butter

1 pound apricots, halved
and pitted

1 teaspoon licorice root powder

1 teaspoon ground cinnamon

¼ teaspoon ground ginger

¼ teaspoon ground cardamom

1 tablespoon maple syrup

Rye has a lovely, sturdy flavor and makes delicious porridge. Soaking it in advance helps release enzymes that make both the grain gentler on your digestive system and its minerals easier for your body to absorb. If you don't care for rye or need a gluten-free alternative, old-fashioned rolled oats work well in this recipe, too. Cooking the porridge in apple juice gives it plenty of sweetness and a pleasant flavor that partners well with apricots and sweet spices. To accommodate the need for soaking the rye flakes, start this recipe the night before you plan to serve it.

---

to make the porridge: Dump the rye in a medium mixing bowl and then pour in enough hot water to cover by 2 inches. Stir in the vinegar and salt and let the rye soak overnight for at least 8 and up to 12 hours.

The next morning, strain the rye in a fine-mesh sieve and then transfer it to a medium saucepan. Cover it with the apple juice, bring it to a boil over medium-high heat, and then immediately turn the heat to medium-low and stir until cooked through, about 10 minutes. Turn off the heat, cover the pot, and keep it warm while you prepare the apricots.

to make the apricots: Warm a wide skillet over medium heat and then add in the ghee. When it melts, add the apricots, licorice, cinnamon, ginger, and cardamom and stir until the fruit begins to soften without losing its form, about 5 minutes. Stir in the maple syrup and turn off the heat.

To serve, ladle the porridge into bowls and top with apricots.

eleuthero

(eleutherococcus senticosus)

Eleuthero grows in low thickets among expansive coniferous trees in the forested mountains of Northeast Asia. The people who live in China and Eastern Russia have used eleuthero for centuries as both food and medicine. They gather its roots and bark in the fall when medicinal compounds in the herb are at their peak. As a food, eleuthero is a source of many minerals, including calcium, phosphorus, magnesium, potassium, and zinc. Beyond its nutritive minerals, the herb's medicinal compounds give it a reputation as a strengthening tonic. Like many medicinal roots, eleuthero tastes slightly sweet and bitter, with woodsy notes.

As an adaptogen, eleuthero has a gentle systemic action that builds resilience against stress. It supports the adrenal glands and has a normalizing effect on the body's stress-response hormones. It also regulates the immune system, strengthening it against potential stressors, such as viruses that cause colds and flu.

As a mild stimulating herb, eleuthero also combats fatigue and enhances stamina. It works well for people who work demanding jobs, athletes, or anyone who needs a sustained energy boost.

Look for responsibly wildcrafted eleuthero root online from retailers specializing in medicinal herbs. You may also find it in the supplement section of your local health food store. It's commonly available in capsules, tinctures, and compound herbal formulas. Buy the dried root or eleuthero powder to minimize additives widely used in capsules.

Using it in the kitchen: Eleuthero is mostly used in medicinal remedies rather than as a culinary herb. Add eleuthero powder to other strong-tasting herbs such as cacao (see page 27) or cinnamon.

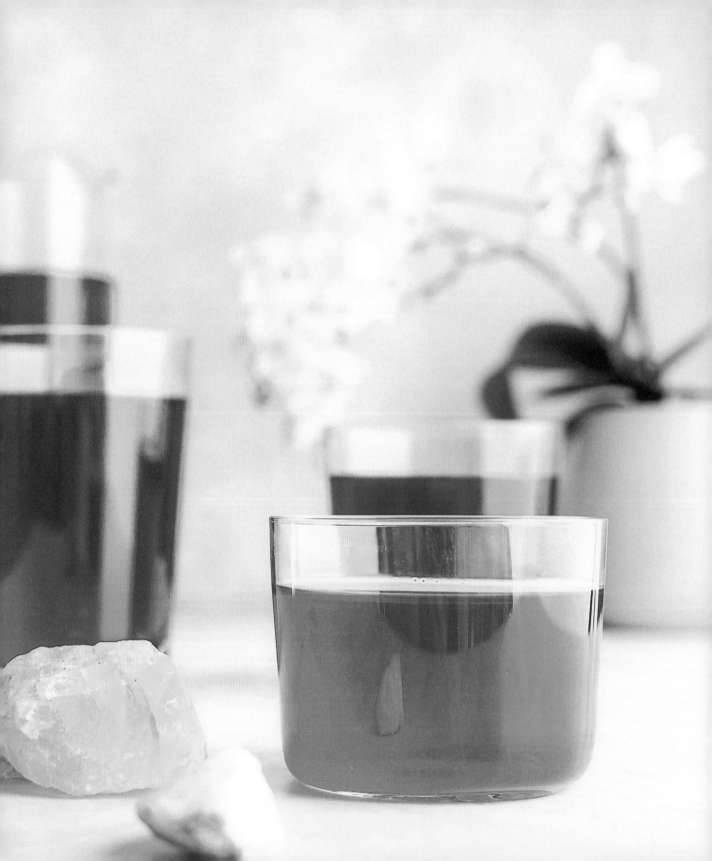

energizing morning elixir

MAKES ABOUT 6 SERVINGS

8 cups cold water

2 tablespoons cut and sifted dried eleuthero root

2 tablespoons dried schisandra berries

1 tablespoon cut and seeded dried rosehips

2 teaspoons cut and sifted dried licorice root

1 (3-inch) knob ginger, coarsely chopped

¼ cup dried hibiscus flowers

A nutritionist I work with, Lydia Joy, shared this recipe with me as an easy way to support adrenal health when you're feeling burnt out from prolonged stress. It's an energizing blend, owing to the eleuthero and licorice root, that's also positively packed with antioxidants and other plant nutrients.

I've tinkered with the recipe over the years, dropping stevia and cinnamon in favor of brilliant red hibiscus and rosehips for added vitamin C. You can make a big batch and store it in the refrigerator for a few days so it's easy to grab in the morning. It's also equally as delicious cold as it is warm. Because it's a stimulating blend of herbs, try sipping it in the morning and nourishing yourself with quieter herbs like passionflower or tulsi in the evening.

In a medium saucepan over medium-high heat, combine the water, eleuthero, schisandra, rosehips, licorice, and ginger, bring to a boil, and then turn down the heat to low and simmer the herbs for about 20 minutes. Turn off the heat completely and then toss in the hibiscus flowers. Cover the pot and let the herbs steep together for 20 minutes more.

Strain the infusion through a fine-mesh sieve into a 2-quart jar, discarding the solids. Drink immediately or seal the jar, label it, and transfer it to the refrigerator. The infusion will keep for about 3 days.

chicory and dandelion latte

MAKES ABOUT 2 SERVINGS

1½ cups cold water

1 tablespoon cut and sifted dried roasted dandelion root

1 tablespoon roasted chicory root granules

2 teaspoons cut and sifted dried eleuthero root

1 vanilla bean, split

1 cup milk

Roasted chicory and dandelion roots (page 154) taste toasty and faintly bitter, almost like coffee. Indeed, the flavors blend so well that chicory root is often added to coffee to give the brew balance and a touch of sweetness, a practice that likely began in Holland before making its way to France, the United Kingdom, southern India, and New Orleans. While it won't replace your coffee, this herbal latte does make a pleasant, nourishing elixir on cold mornings. Dandelion and chicory support your liver, while eleuthero builds stamina and fortifies your body against day-to-day stress.

If you find it's too bitter, swirl in a spoonful of coconut sugar or maple syrup to your liking before whisking in hot milk. Whole milk works well in this recipe because it foams so readily, but you can use a dairy-free alternative if you like, or serve the infusion straight, without any milk at all. You can also double the recipe and store the infusion in the refrigerator. Just warm it up and add milk when you're ready to serve. The infusion will start to lose potency after about 3 days.

In a small saucepan over medium-high heat, combine the water, dandelion, chicory, eleuthero, and vanilla bean, bring to a boil, and then immediately turn the heat down to low. Simmer, uncovered, for about 20 minutes, then turn off the heat and strain the infusion through a fine-mesh strainer into a 1-quart Mason jar.

Wipe out the saucepan, return it to the stove, and then pour in the milk. Heat the milk until pleasantly hot and steaming (about 160°F), whisking it constantly. Pour the hot milk into the herbal infusion and serve right away.

rhodiola

(rhodiola rosea)

Rhodiola is an arctic succulent that grows in little clumps of blue-green leaves. In the summertime, it blossoms with clusters of tiny, sunshine-yellow flowers. The plant's ruddy root smells vaguely of roses, and it holds a sacred medicinal and powerful ability to energize, nourish, and lift the spirit.

Folks who live in Russia and Scandinavia have used rhodiola for centuries as both food and medicine. They prize the herb for its exceptional ability to energize the body and fortify the spirit against the stress of long, cold winters. In herbal folk medicine, rhodiola was used to improve stamina and ease fatigue.

Rhodiola strengthens your body's response to stress and can give you a boost of energy when you need it. Studies have also found that rhodiola extracts ease stress-induced depression, uplifting a melancholic mood, and are generally well tolerated by the people who take it. That's likely because it supports the hypothalamus, adrenal, and pituitary glands, which govern the body's stress-response system. Additionally, rhodiola influences chemicals in your brain called neurotransmitters that regulate mood. The herb also stimulates and protects the nervous system and can be an ally to brain health as you age.

Use rhodiola when you need a quick shot of energy or when you need to concentrate. You can also use rhodiola over a more extended period for its stress-reducing and mood-boosting effects.

Purchase dried rhodiola root, tinctures, and powders from high-quality medicinal herb providers. Increasing interest in adaptogens in recent years has led to the overharvesting of wild rhodiola. Look for responsibly farmed or ethically wildcrafted options. Because it is an energizing herb, take it early in the day when your body will benefit from the boost, and try calming herbs such as chamomile (see page 217) or California poppy (see page 210) in the evening.

Using it in the kitchen: Take rhodiola tea before breakfast as an energizing and revitalizing elixir. Use rhodiola powder blended with other herbs to season your foods, but use it judiciously lest its potent, bitter flavor overpower the dishes you make.

bircher muesli with rhodiola-strawberry syrup

MAKES 4 SERVINGS

rhodiola-strawberry syrup

1 teaspoon cut and sifted dried rhodiola root

1 vanilla bean, split

1½ cups cold water

3 tablespoons dried rose petals

1 pound strawberries, hulled and halved

½ cup honey

muesli

2 apples with skin intact, cored and coarsely grated

1 cup sprouted rolled oats

1 cup plain full-fat yogurt

½ cup heavy cream

¼ teaspoon fine sea salt

½ pound strawberries, hulled and halved

½ cup coarsely chopped raw hazelnuts

When my family and I visited Switzerland several years ago on the hunt for traditional alpine foods, we ate muesli with freshly made raw yogurt almost every morning. Muesli is an Alpine dish popularized by an early twentieth-century Swiss doctor named Maximilian Bircher-Benner, who served it to his patients with the hope that it might strengthen their bodies, support their digestion, and speed healing. While not originally intended as a breakfast, muesli makes an excellent and nutritious start to the day. Bircher-Benner's original version calls for honey and condensed milk, but I like to build flavor with herbal syrup.

This recipe takes a little advanced planning, but it pays off with an easy, nourishing breakfast. So make the syrup up to 3 days in advance and begin mixing the muesli the night before, allowing it to soak overnight, so that it's ready first thing in the morning.

to make the syrup: In a small saucepan over medium-high heat, combine the rhodiola root and vanilla bean, cover with the cold water, and bring to a boil. Turn the heat down to medium and simmer, uncovered, until the liquid is reduced by half, about 15 minutes. Turn off the heat and toss in the rose petals. Cover the pot and let steep for about 5 minutes.

Strain the liquid through a fine-mesh sieve into a food processor or blender, discarding the solids. Toss in the strawberries and honey and process until smooth. Pour the syrup into a pint-sized jar, seal, label, and refrigerate until you're ready to serve the muesli. The syrup will keep for about 5 days.

to make the muesli: The night before you plan to serve the muesli for breakfast, in a large bowl, stir together the apples, oats, yogurt, cream, and salt. Cover tightly and set it aside in a cool spot on your countertop.

The next morning, stir the muesli once more and then spoon equal portions into four bowls. Sprinkle the muesli with strawberries and hazelnuts and drizzle with the Rhodiola-Strawberry syrup.

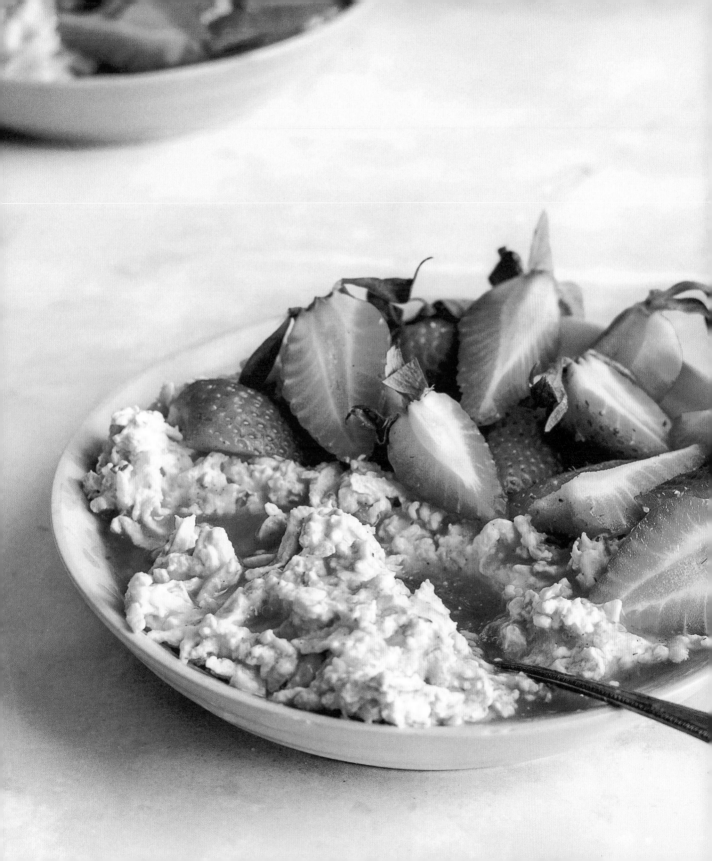

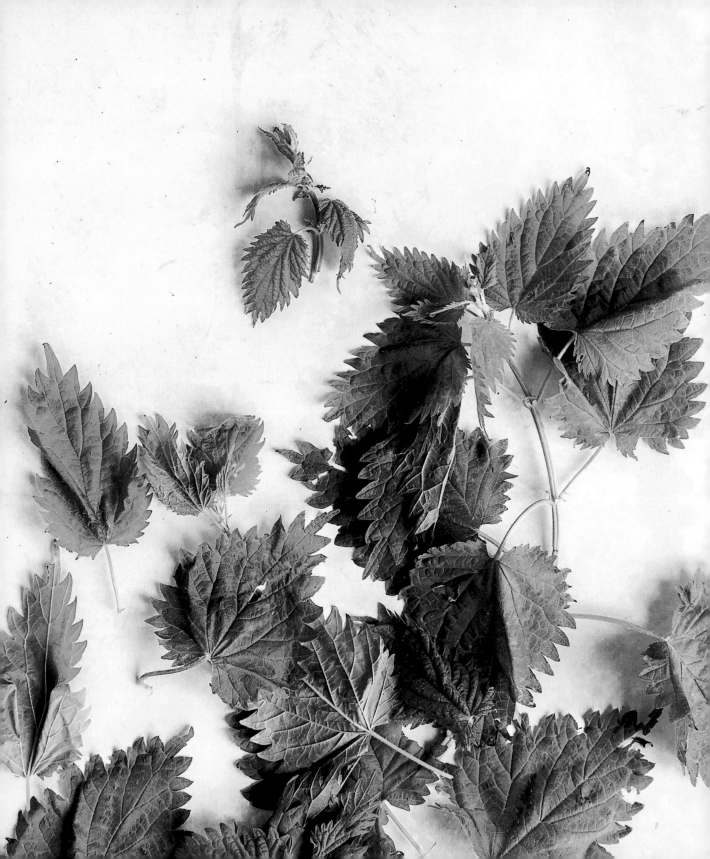

stinging nettle
(urtica dioica)

Stinging nettle grows wild in temperate climates throughout the world. You'll find it springing up in patches along alleyways, behind homes, at the edges of streams, and on the forest floor. It looks innocuous enough, with its tall stems and serrated green leaves, but if you brush against the plant, your skin will erupt in small, painfully itchy bumps. The tiny hairs that adhere to the underside of the nettle leaf serve as a warning to would-be predators, and they give nettle its characteristic sting.

Stinging nettle itself is a profoundly nutritious herb and is exceptionally rich in vitamins A and K, as well as magnesium and calcium. It also contains vitamin B_6, phosphorus, iron, manganese, and potassium. Its rich array of minerals makes the leaves excellent for remineralizing the body. Its deep nutrition offers gentle, grounding energy, and you can enjoy it daily as a simple, nourishing tonic.

Beyond its nutritive qualities, stinging nettle fights systemic inflammation. Its anti-inflammatory compounds support the heart, kidneys, and adrenal glands. As an adrenal tonic, the herb helps your body build resilience against stress, giving you supportive energy and stamina to get you through your day.

In European traditions, herbalists used stinging nettle in blood sugar–balancing tisanes and for natural allergy relief. The anti-inflammatory compounds in stinging nettle, as well as its nourishing minerals and fiber, stabilize blood sugar and can help promote metabolic health. Similarly, stinging nettle acts as a natural antihistamine, and many people drink inky nettle infusions during allergy season.

While the whole stinging nettle plant is edible, the young, tender leaves are both particularly nutritious and delicious. They have a salty quality from the plentiful minerals they contain, and a flavor similar to spinach. Find the leafy tops fresh in spring or at farmers' markets and specialty grocers. The leaves are also available dried, but make sure to purchase organic or ethically wildcrafted options.

Using it in the kitchen: Wear gloves and long sleeves when handling fresh nettle leaves, because they can sting. If you puree raw stinging nettle leaves, the herb will lose its sting. Raw stinging nettle makes a delicious pesto, and you can also add it to smoothies. Cook the leaves as you would any other tender leafy green.

baked eggs with nettle–pumpkin seed pesto

MAKES 4 SERVINGS

4 teaspoons salted butter, melted

8 eggs

1½ cups tightly packed fresh stinging nettle leaves

½ cup tightly packed fresh flat-leaf parsley

1 jalapeño chile, seeded and finely chopped

2 garlic cloves, chopped

¼ cup pumpkin seeds

1 teaspoon fine sea salt

Juice of 1 lemon

¼ cup extra-virgin olive oil

Baked eggs, their yolks all yellow and jammy, make a beautiful and simple breakfast. In the springtime when both local eggs and young, tender stinging nettle leaves are available, I like to make this dish. It's easy, nutrient-dense, and speaks to the season. Bright green nettle–pumpkin seed pesto, spiked with garlic and jalapeño, offers a pleasant contrast to the creaminess of baked eggs.

While fresh stinging nettle can irritate the skin, don't let that put you off from making this raw nettle pesto. Like both drying and cooking, pureeing the plant's leaves neutralizes the compounds that give them their sting, so you can still enjoy stinging nettle fresh in this recipe, where its taste is marvelously green.

Preheat the oven to 350°F and brush four 6-ounce ramekins with 1 teaspoon of melted butter each.

Crack two eggs into each ramekin and then tuck them into the oven to bake for 15 to 18 minutes, until the yolk is set to your liking.

While the eggs bake, in a food processor or high-speed blender, combine the nettles (see page 43 on safe handling), parsley, jalapeño, garlic, pumpkin seeds, salt, lemon juice, and olive oil. Puree until smooth and transfer to a small bowl.

Pull the eggs out of the oven, spoon the nettle pesto over them, and serve immediately. Any extra pesto will keep for up to 5 days in an airtight container in the refrigerator.

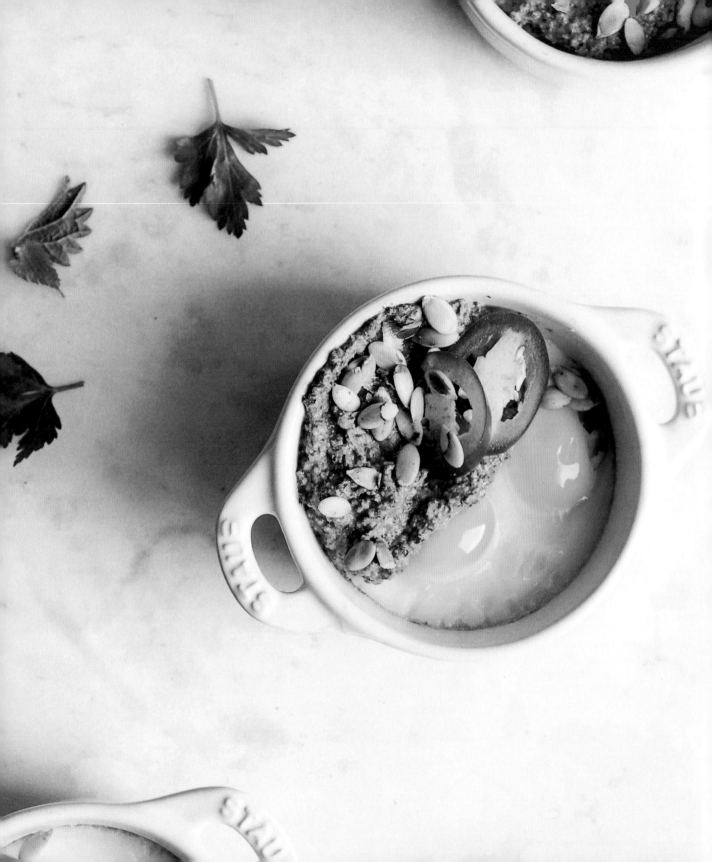

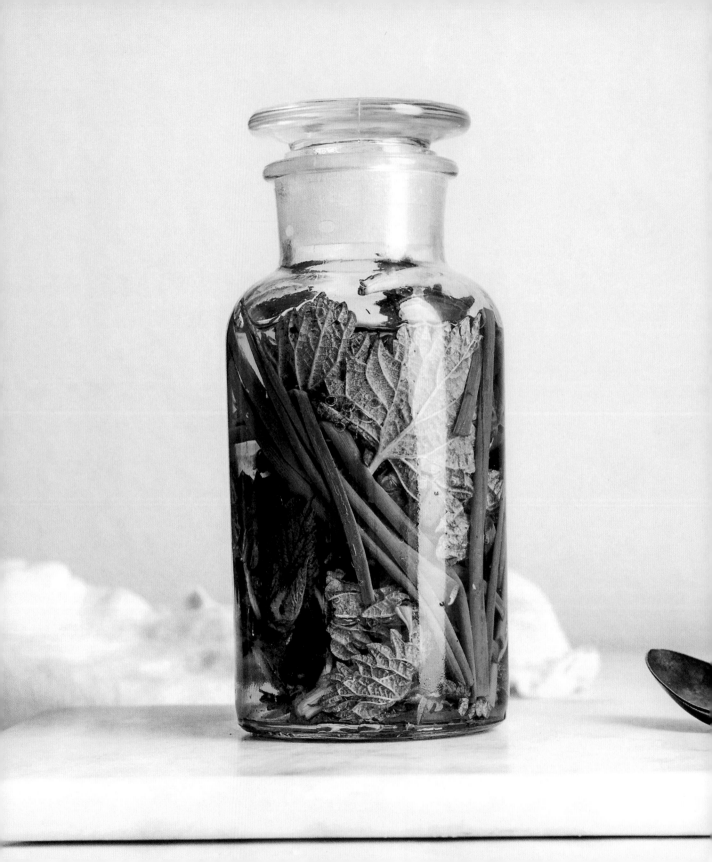

nettle chive vinegar

MAKES ABOUT 3 CUPS

1 cup coarsely chopped fresh
stinging nettle leaves

½ cup chopped fresh chives

3 cups white wine vinegar

Stinging nettle and chives are at their peak in the springtime when the greens are young and tender. You can find both at many farmers' markets if you don't grow or forage for them (in the case of stinging nettles) yourself.

Herbal vinegars excel at extracting an herb's beneficial compounds efficiently and deliciously. If you can fill a jar and remember to shake it daily, you can make herbal vinegars. This herb-infused vinegar has a mild green flavor touched by just the right hint of chives. I love it with olive oil served over the Breakfast Salad with Lox and Herbs (page 48), but you can use it in place of white wine or apple cider vinegar in just about any savory recipe.

Spoon the nettles (see page 43 on safe handling) and chives into a 1-quart jar with a tight-fitting lid and cover them with the vinegar. Seal the jar with a plastic or other nonmetal lid, label it, and tuck it into a dark cupboard away from direct light and heat, shaking it daily for at least 1 month and up to 6 weeks.

Strain the vinegar through a fine-mesh sieve into a 1-quart Mason jar, discarding the solids. Seal the jar with a plastic or nonmetal lid, label it, and store it in a cupboard away from direct light and heat for up to 6 months.

breakfast salad with lox and herbs

MAKES 4 SERVINGS

2 teaspoons caraway seeds

2 teaspoons nigella seeds

1 teaspoon celery seeds

4 cups loosely packed baby arugula

¼ cup loosely packed flat-leaf parsley leaves

2 Persian cucumbers, thinly sliced

2 cups cherry tomatoes, halved

1 shallot, thinly sliced

3 ounces wild-caught salmon lox

2 tablespoons capers

Extra-virgin olive oil for serving

Nettle Chive Vinegar (page 47) for serving

I love to start the day with a big breakfast salad brimming with greens, vegetables, and big flavors. Toasted caraway, nigella, and other spices bring their delicious aromatic qualities to this salad, while capers, cucumbers, and fresh herbs add a little liveliness. While the salad is plenty filling on its own, you can also serve it alongside toasted whole-grain sourdough bread and a poached egg for something a little more substantial.

In a 10-inch cast-iron skillet over medium-high heat, toss in the caraway, nigella, and celery seeds. Toast for about 3 minutes, stirring constantly, until fragrant, and then spoon them into a small bowl, letting them cool while you prepare the salad.

In a large bowl, toss the arugula with the parsley until well mixed and then arrange the greens on four plates. Arrange the cucumbers, tomatoes, shallot, and salmon over the greens and then sprinkle with capers and the toasted spices. Drizzle with the olive oil and vinegar to your liking and serve.

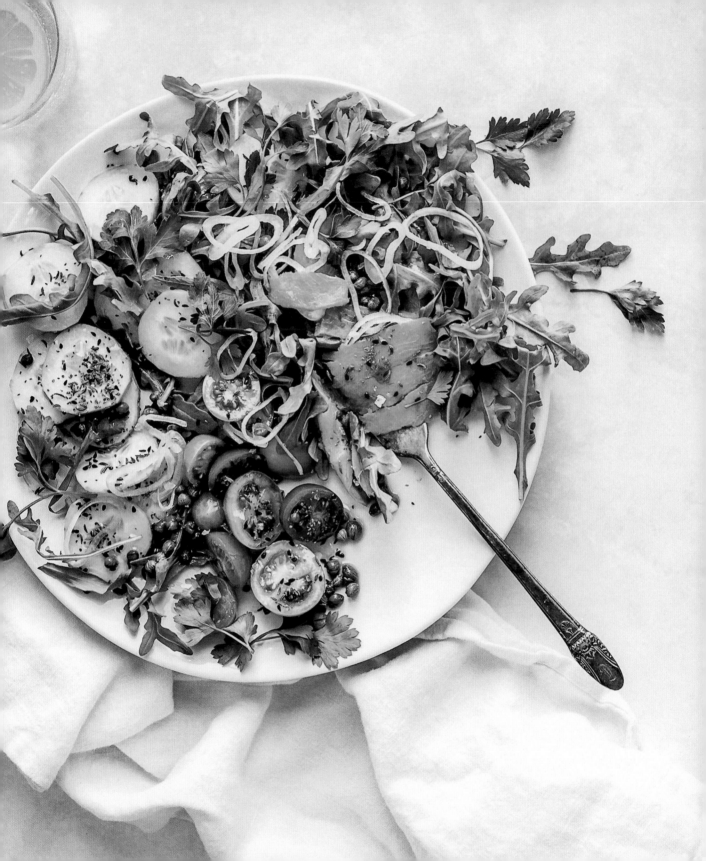

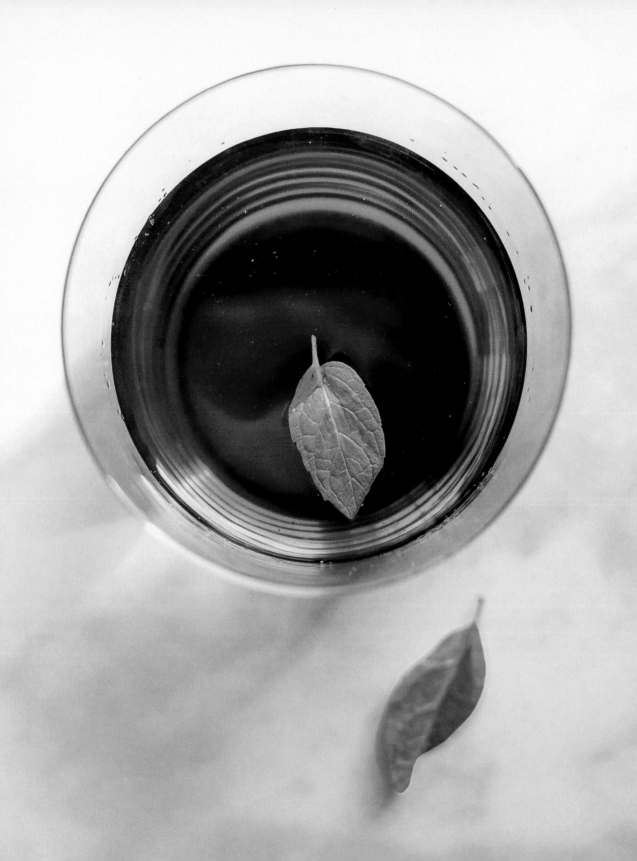

nettle mint infusion

8 cups water

1 cup dried cut and sifted stinging nettle

½ cup dried spearmint

While you can drink nourishing, mineral-rich infusions throughout the day, drinking them first thing in the morning has an energizing effect. It's a simple act of self-care that can set the tone for the day, because even if everything else feels as if it's falling apart, you've at least done yourself a good turn first thing in the morning.

Stinging nettle is an extraordinary, nutritive herb, and infusions like this one help hydrate and remineralize the body while also supporting the adrenal glands. You can enjoy the infusion hot or chilled over ice.

In medium saucepan over high heat, bring the water to a boil. While the water comes to temperature, toss the nettles and spearmint into a 2-quart Mason jar. Pour the boiling water over the herbs, seal tightly, and let them steep in the hot water for at least 4 and up to 12 hours.

Strain the infusion through a fine-mesh sieve into a clean 2-quart Mason jar. Enjoy right away or seal, label, and store it in the refrigerator for up to 3 days.

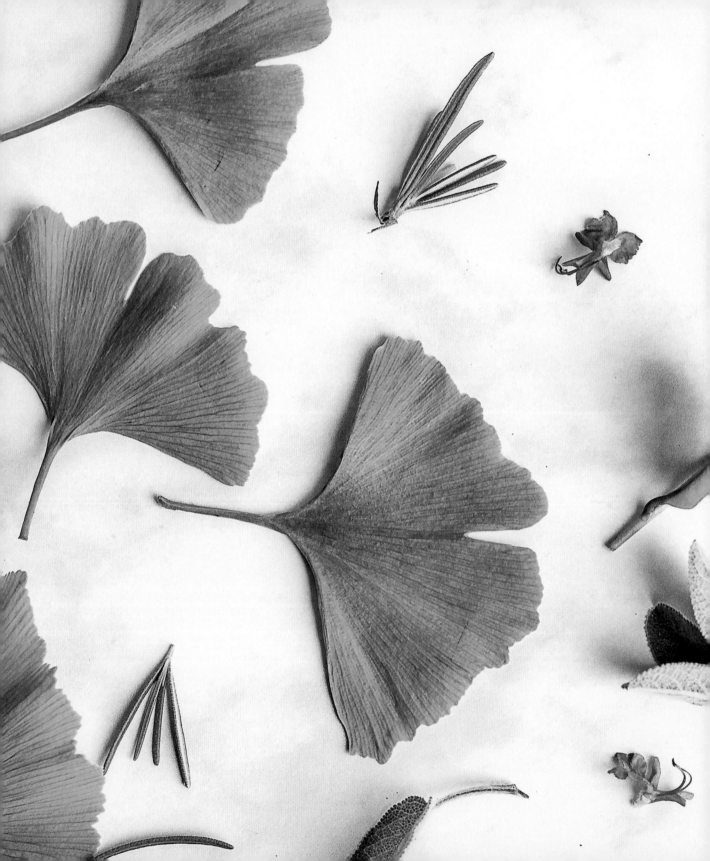

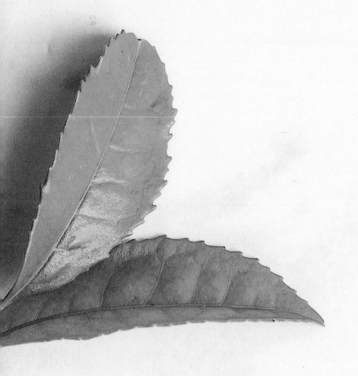

CHAPTER 3

herbs for mental clarity

Herbs have a gentle but powerful effect on the body, especially when used with time, intention, and consistency. They cool inflammation, reduce stress, and many promote mental clarity, cognitive health, and memory. Their effects can be particularly valuable for students, people who work mentally taxing jobs, and those of us who want to keep our minds sharp and agile as we age.

You might find that breathing in the aroma of freshly cut rosemary better prepares you for study, or that you enjoy a clearer mind when you drink green tea regularly. Herbalists celebrate the ability of specific herbs to support memory, concentration, and mental clarity. These herbs fold themselves into the healing traditions throughout the world, and researchers are now investigating just what it is within these herbs that give them their reputation as potent botanicals for brain health and cognition. Often, the work of current researchers supports what traditional healers have known for some time: herbs hold powerful medicine.

Herbs support mental clarity, memory, and concentration in a few ways. Most herbs are rich in antioxidants, which cool the inflammation that stresses your body's cells. Others, like tea, have a slightly stimulating effect on the nervous system, increasing focus. Sage and other similar herbs contain compounds that work with neurotransmitters (chemical messengers within your brain) that are responsible for mood, memory, and concentration. Most herbs work in a combination of ways rather than singly, combat inflammation while also stimulating the nervous system or enhancing the performance of neurotransmitters.

Enjoy these herbs throughout the day, but if you're sensitive to caffeine, limit the more stimulating herbs to the morning.

herbs to enhance memory and concentration

Energizing herbs: Stimulating nervines, such as tea (see page 57) and coffee, can excite the nerves and energize the mind, increasing concentration. Many also open up the blood vessels, which encourages blood flow to the brain. Some may increase jitteriness or keep you awake if you take them too late in the day.

Memory enhancers: Nootropic herbs support the brain, improving memory and focus. Herbs such as saffron (see page 78), rosemary (see page 65), and sage (see page 72) are rich in antioxidants, which combat inflammation. They also contain various compounds that work within the brain to improve memory, concentration, and even mood.

Stress busters: Adaptogens, herbs that support your body's ability to adapt to stress, complement memory enhancers and energizing herbs to support brain health. Reishi (see page 104), tulsi (see page 162), and licorice root (see page 31), and similar herbs fortify the body against stress that can impact the brain.

Anti-inflammatory herbs: Antioxidant-rich herbs calm inflammation throughout your body. The potent compounds within these herbs can scavenge free radicals and support cellular health.

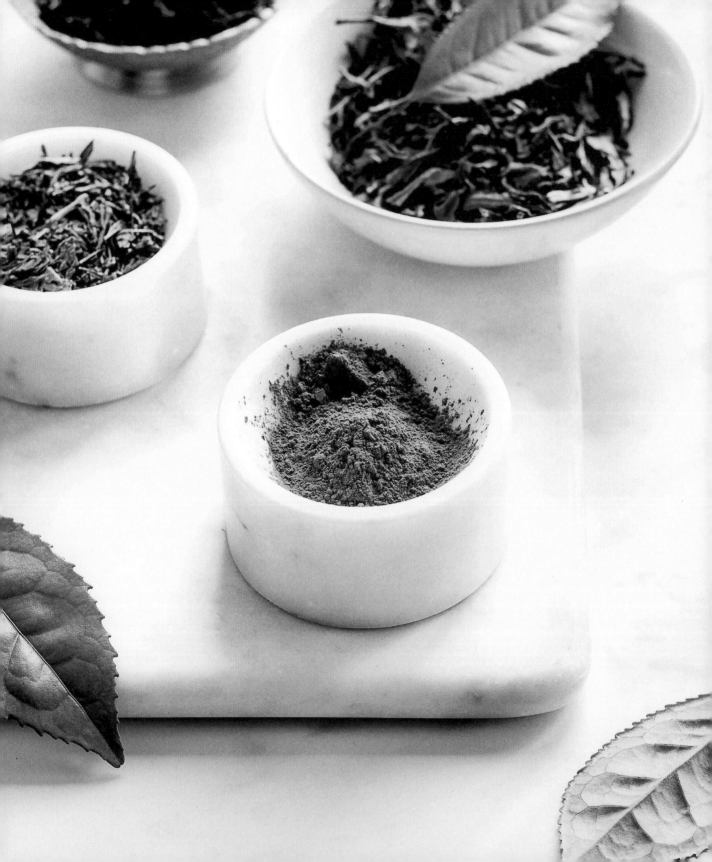

tea

(camellia sinensis)

Tea is an evergreen shrub with glossy dark green leaves. It's the smallest tea buds that are most prized, as they carry the best flavor, both delicate and pronounced. That's because the young buds are also the most abundant source of medicinal compounds within the plant. They're extraordinarily high in the antioxidants and anti-inflammatory compounds that give tea its reputation as an elixir of health and longevity.

After picking, tea producers process the leaves to develop their distinct aromas and flavors. White and green teas are the most delicate and the least processed. After agricultural workers pluck the tender young buds, they allow them to whither before drying in order to produce white tea. For green tea, tender young leaves are first steamed or roasted before drying. Darker teas with more robust flavor, such as oolong and black tea, undergo varying degrees of oxidation, with pu'erh being fermented.

While each variety of tea has distinct benefits and flavor, green and white teas boast particularly high antioxidant content. In addition to antioxidants, tea is also high in an amino acid called L-theanine. This compound promotes an alert relaxation without causing drowsiness. It also supports memory and concentration without causing jitteriness. Tea's ability to support peaceful focus makes it a great choice when you need to concentrate, finish a project, or focus on work and studies.

Tea's high antioxidant content also means that it helps your body build resilience against oxidative stress and inflammation—the root cause of many chronic diseases. Drinking tea, specifically green and white tea, is also linked to better heart and metabolic health.

Matcha is particularly high in beneficial compounds, and that's because a few weeks before harvest, farmers shade the growing plants. This practice stresses the plants. In response, they increase their production of certain micronutrients such as chlorophyll, catechins, and other antioxidants, as well as amino acids such as L-theanine. As a result, matcha is a concentrated source of these nutrients and has a stronger medicinal effect than most brewed teas.

Look for loose-leaf teas where possible, as they tend to be higher quality than bagged teas, and ceremonial-grade matcha, which comes in vivid green powder form and tends to be the best quality in terms of taste and medicinal value. Keep in mind that tea, like many plants, absorbs fluoride and heavy metals from the soil in which it grows, and they can end up in your cup. While fluoride occurs naturally in soil, it and heavy metals are often used in pesticides and other agriculture inputs applied to many plants. Buy organically grown tea, where possible, to minimize both heavy metals and pesticide residue.

Buy fair-trade options where possible, too. Tea pickers are overwhelmingly women and girls and are often subject to sex-based violence and poor living conditions on the estates where they work. Low wages, inadequate food, and unsanitary shelters contribute to malnutrition and disease in workers. By purchasing fair-trade and ethically produced tea, you actively change these pathways and contribute to a food system that values workers, ecology, and health.

Using it in the kitchen: The easiest way to enjoy tea is as a hot-water infusion. White and green tea benefit from a lower water temperature than black tea. Lower water temperature gives the more delicate notes in these teas an opportunity to bloom. You can also blend tea powders, such as matcha, into other foods as a seasoning.

How to steep tea: Different types of tea benefit from different brewing techniques. Delicate green teas benefit from low temperatures and brief steeping or they become bitter, while dark black tea can withstand higher temperatures and longer steep times. When you steep your tea at the appropriate temperature and keep an eye on the time, you allow the full flavor of the tea to blossom.

Type of Tea	Water Temperature	Timing
White	194°F	2 to 3 minutes
Green	175°F	2 to 4 minutes
Oolong	185°F	3 to 5 minutes
Black	205°F	3 to 5 minutes

iced sencha with spearmint and ginkgo

MAKES ABOUT 6 SERVINGS

1 tablespoon dried spearmint

1 tablespoon dried ginkgo leaf

8 cups boiling water

2 tablespoons sencha tea

Thinly sliced lemon for serving

Sencha tastes deliciously green with a slightly savory undertone owing to its high level of amino acids, particularly L-theanine, which promotes a sense of calm but focused concentration. It blends beautifully with the soft, bitter notes of ginkgo, while spearmint (see page 146) gives the blend both clarity and a harmonious, activating energy. Pour the cooled tea over ice and sip it on days when you need both refreshment and greater mental clarity—ginkgo (see page 63) and sencha make great companions for study and difficult mental work.

Herbs like ginkgo and spearmint need higher temperatures and longer steep times to release their flavor and medicine, but true tea (*Camellia sinensis*) benefits from a gentler brewing technique, or it can become bitter and overly tannic. Instead of adding all the herbs to hot water all at once, which might burn the sencha or weaken the ginkgo and mint, try using a two-fold brewing technique. First, you'll steep the sturdier herbs in boiling water, and when it cools to the lower temperature favored for green tea, swirl in the sencha. As a result, the ginkgo and mint release their full flavor and the more fragile sencha retains its delicate notes without tasting bitter.

Spoon the spearmint and ginkgo into a 2-quart Mason jar and cover them with the boiling water. Let steep until it reaches about 175°F and then stir in the sencha with a long-handled spoon. Continue to steep for about 3 minutes more, then strain the liquid into a clean 2-quart Mason jar and transfer it to the refrigerator to cool completely.

Serve over ice with a slice of lemon and use it all within 3 days.

melon in matcha-honey syrup

¼ cup honey

¼ cup water

2 tablespoons matcha tea

1 small honeydew melon
(about 2 pounds)

½ cup chopped fresh mint

Melon's sweetness marries well with the bitter, savory notes of matcha tea. This recipe calls for honeydew, which you can find at just about any grocery store. If you're lucky enough to have a farmers' market nearby, you can swap honeydew for heirloom varietals like Charentais, Petit Gris de Rennes, or the Rajasthan Honey Melon. They ripen in late summer, with a concentrated sweetness and more resonant flavor than most melons you'll find in the grocery store, which are primarily bred to withstand lengthy and arduous transport rather than for flavor.

I like to serve melons in matcha-honey syrup in the summertime for breakfast, alongside yogurt dressed with pumpkin seeds and almonds. Matcha has an energy-boosting effect, making it a lovely choice to start your day. This recipe also makes an easy snack or simple dessert. You can use the matcha syrup on other fruits, too, and it pairs well with blackberries.

In a small saucepan over medium-low heat, whisk together the honey and water until the honey dissolves completely. Turn off the heat and stir in the matcha powder, then transfer the syrup to the refrigerator to cool while you prepare the melon.

Scrub the melon under hot water and then dry it with a kitchen towel. Cut it in half, then scoop out the seeds and discard them. Slice into thin wedges, about ½ inch thick, and arrange them on a serving dish. Scatter the mint over the melon and then drizzle it all with matcha-honey syrup.

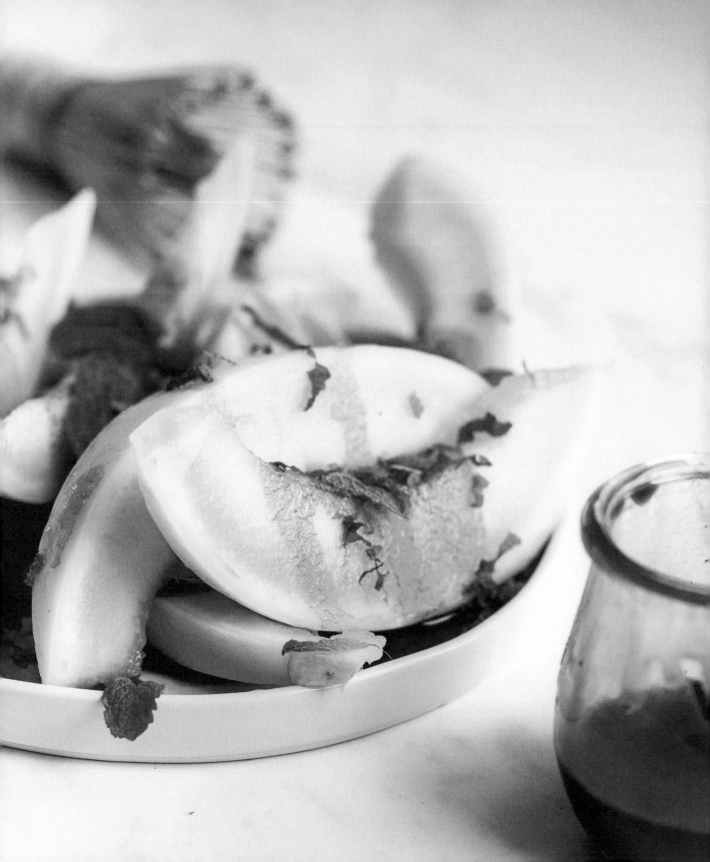

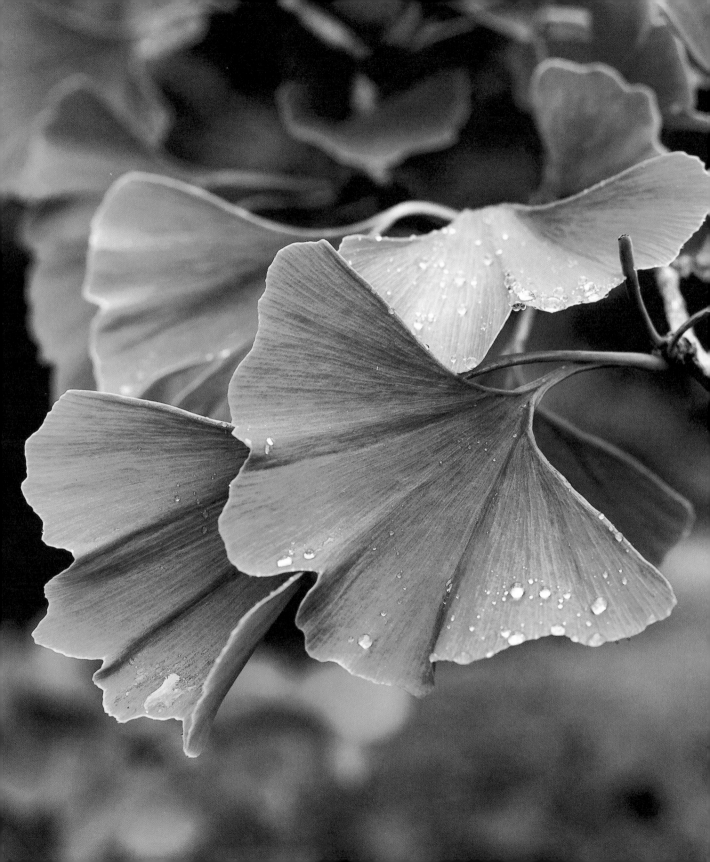

ginkgo
(ginkgo biloba)

In the autumn, ginkgo trees turn a glorious, breathtaking gold. Then, when a hard freeze hits, they drop their feathery leaves seemingly all at once. A symbol of tenacity and longevity, the trees can survive for more than a thousand years. While they're native to southeastern China, you won't find them in the wild any longer, but you can often see some of the oldest trees in Chinese and Japanese monasteries.

Practitioners of traditional Chinese medicine have used ginkgo leaves for millennia, primarily to strengthen the lungs. Current research into ginkgo's benefits supports this use, particularly for asthma. Perhaps what ginkgo is best known for is its ability to promote brain health and cognition, especially as you age. Ginkgo also sharpens mental focus, bringing clarity to those under chronic stress.

Ginkgo is rich in antioxidants, and it's these protective compounds that help reduce oxidative stress in your body and counteract free radicals. Further, specific compounds unique to ginkgo encourage the bronchial tubes in your lungs to open up so you can breathe easier. Those same compounds also promote better blood flow throughout your body, including your brain, which may account for some of the herb's benefits.

You can find ginkgo in capsules, tinctures, and extracts, but the dried leaf, which is harvested in late summer, is best to keep on hand.

Using it in the kitchen: Ginkgo supplements are popular, but you can use the plant as you would other dry leafy herbs. Use ginkgo in teas and infusions or toss some into a soup stock where its tart and faintly sweet taste can bring both flavor and nutrition.

three-herb ghee

2 cups unsalted butter, cubed

¼ cup dried ginkgo leaves

1 tablespoon dried sage

1 tablespoon dried rosemary

My friend Sandeep Agarwal, who runs Pure Indian Foods with his wife, Nalini, makes the most delicious herbal ghee, some infused with medicinal herbs such as ashwagandha (see page 192) and shatavari, and others with aromatic herbs such as cardamom (see page 135) or fennel (see page 141). Inspired by his work, I've enjoyed making my own with local butter and herbs from my own garden such as this version, which includes ginkgo, sage, and rosemary.

Butter is a beautiful and practical vehicle for both medicinal and culinary herbs. The warmth of hot butter encourages herbs to release the compounds that give the plants both their characteristic flavors and benefits. Making ghee is a gentle process of separating the milk solids in butter from pure butterfat. As you melt the butter, it will release its foam, which consists of various proteins and sugars naturally found in cream. Skimming away the foam, and then filtering the hot butter for good measure, leaves nothing but the pure golden butterfat with its rich, almost nutty flavor. Because ghee is pure butterfat, it not only captures the flavor of herbs but also preserves it for months. Use herbal ghee in place of butter, olive oil, or other cooking fats to fry eggs in the morning, pop popcorn for a snack, or roast root vegetables as a side dish.

In a wide skillet over low heat, heat the butter until it melts and begins to foam. Skim off any foam with a skimmer or a spoon and discard it.

Stir the ginkgo, sage, and rosemary into the hot butter and continue cooking over low heat for about 20 minutes, until the remaining milk solids sink and begin to brown. Remove any additional foam as it forms.

Set a double layer of cheesecloth into a fine-mesh sieve and strain the butter through the cheesecloth into a pint-sized Mason jar, discarding the solids.

Let the ghee cool completely. Seal, label, and store the jar in a dark cupboard away from light and heat for up to 3 months or in the refrigerator for up to 1 year.

rosemary

(salvia rosmarinus)

Rosemary is a spiny shrub with needlelike leaves and a woodsy, herbaceous perfume. If you've ever brushed up against a rosemary bush in the garden on a warm day, you know how its tenacious aroma lingers on your skin. That distinct perfume comes from a wide array of volatile oils that also give the herb its resonant and unmistakable flavor.

Rosemary's resonant perfume and penetrating flavor also signify the presence of various medicinal plant compounds. As a bitter herb, rosemary stimulates and supports the digestive system, particularly the liver and gallbladder. Further, it also calms the nerves and complements similar herbs to uplift a worn spirit. The herb's tranquil qualities also make it an excellent tonic for the heart, and it helps increase blood flow to the brain as well. Because rosemary encourages blood flow, which benefits your heart and brain, it can also stimulate and increase menstrual flow. This action makes rosemary helpful if you're suffering from cramps related to your cycle, but if you're pregnant, it's best to avoid eating large concentrated doses of rosemary as well as rosemary infusions and tinctures.

Herbalists have long used rosemary to boost mental clarity and increase memory and concentration. Antioxidants and anti-inflammatory compounds in rosemary reduce oxidative stress and support brain health and cognition. For this reason, it's an excellent herb for students and people who work mentally taxing jobs, and it can support people as they age.

While you can find both fresh and dried rosemary in most grocery stores, opt for fresh whenever possible. Rosemary's volatile oils dissipate quickly when dried. It also grows well in a variety of climates without much attention, so you can add it to your garden or tuck it into a pot on your patio. That way you'll always have a ready supply.

Using it in the kitchen: Rosemary partners well with roasted meats and root vegetables, as its uplifting aroma lends a little brightness to these earthy foods. Tuck a sprig or two into a pot of soup or sprinkle chopped rosemary over your vegetables before you roast them in the oven. When using the herb therapeutically, try a tisane, infusion, or even a tincture for a more concentrated dose.

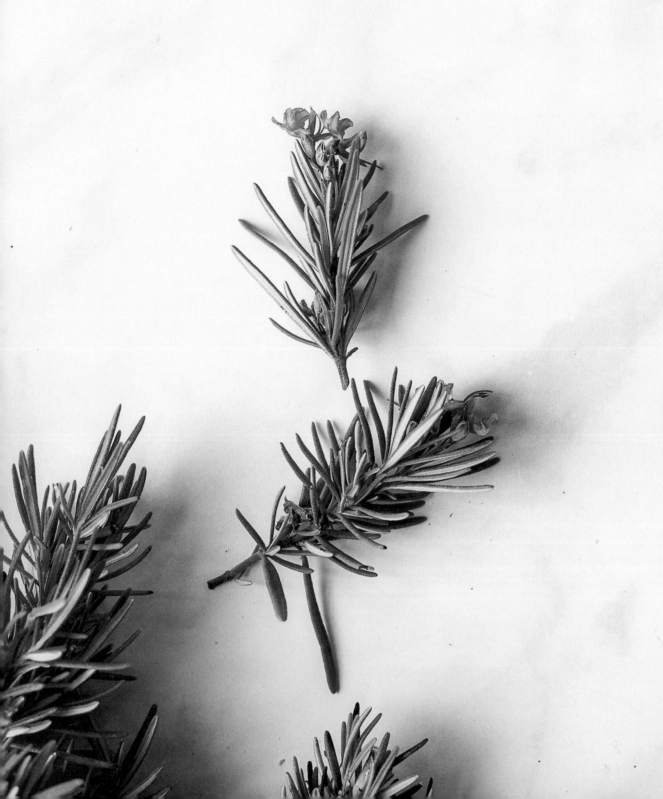

rosemary and sage oil

MAKES ABOUT 1 CUP

¼ cup dried rosemary

2 tablespoons dried sage

1 cup extra-virgin olive oil

Rosemary and sage belong together. Both build upon each other's aroma, creating deeper flavor. Use this oil to build flavor into other dishes. Swirl it into a hot skillet with a spoonful of chopped fresh garlic. Drizzle it over vegetables just before you toss them into the oven to roast, or whisk it into a vinaigrette for your next salad.

Infusing oils with herbs is an exercise in delayed gratification. While it takes only a moment of active time in the kitchen to make an herb-infused oil, it takes a month of slow, gentle extraction for the herbs to yield their aroma and medicine. This passive process requires patience on your part but, fortunately, little effort. Some herbalists speed the process with heat, but I prefer to tuck the herbs into the cupboard, letting time extract their benefits rather than force.

Using a mortar and pestle, your fingertips, a spice grinder, or food processor, coarsely grind the rosemary and sage to break up the cell walls and activate the herbs—taking care to stop before they turn to powder.

Spoon the herbs into a 1-pint jar with a tight-fitting lid and cover them with the extra-virgin olive oil. Seal the jar tightly and then shake it vigorously to distribute the herbs. Set the jar in a warm spot in your kitchen and shake it once a day for 1 month.

Strain the infused oil through a fine-mesh sieve into a 1-pint Mason jar, discarding the solids. Seal, label, and store the jar in a cupboard away from direct light and heat for up to 1 year.

roasted butternut squash soup with sage and rosemary

2 medium butternut squash (about 3 pounds each)

3 tablespoons extra-virgin olive oil

1 medium yellow onion, coarsely chopped

4 garlic cloves, coarsely chopped

2 teaspoons fine sea salt

¼ cup loosely packed chopped fresh sage

2 tablespoons minced fresh rosemary

2 bay leaves

8 cups chicken bone broth or vegetable stock

Rosemary and Sage Oil (page 67) for drizzling

1 lemon, cut into 6 wedges

In the wintertime, when squash is abundant and cheap, I make this soup weekly. Rosemary and lemon balance the earthy sweetness of butternut squash. It's simple enough to make a big batch and then keep it handy for easy lunches throughout the week.

While you make the soup, enjoy the sensory experience of working with rosemary. Just the act of crushing its needlelike leaves between your fingertips releases its scent. Smelling that aroma alone is not only a pleasant sensorial experience, but it also helps enhance memory and concentration.

Preheat the oven to 400°F and line a rimmed baking sheet with parchment paper.

Slice the squash in half lengthwise and then scoop away the seeds with a spoon. Set the squash on the prepared baking sheet, cut-side down, and transfer it to the oven. Let it roast for at least 30 minutes, until it yields easily when you pierce the skin with a fork.

Set the squash on the counter and let it cool until it's comfortable enough to handle. Then scoop its flesh into a bowl, discarding the skin.

In a Dutch oven set over medium heat, warm the olive oil and then toss in the onion and garlic. Stir for 2 to 3 minutes until the onion and garlic are coated with oil and then sprinkle them with the salt. Drop in the sage and rosemary and continue cooking for 1 to 2 minutes more, allowing the herbs to release their perfume.

Spoon the roasted butternut squash over the onions and garlic and then pour in the broth. Turn down the heat to medium-low and simmer, uncovered, for 15 minutes.

Finish the soup by turning off the heat and then pureeing it until smooth using an immersion blender. If you're using an upright blender, puree the soup in batches taking care to fill the blender only one-third full with each batch.

Ladle the soup into six bowls, drizzle with Rosemary and Sage Oil, and squeeze in a wedge of lemon. Serve warm.

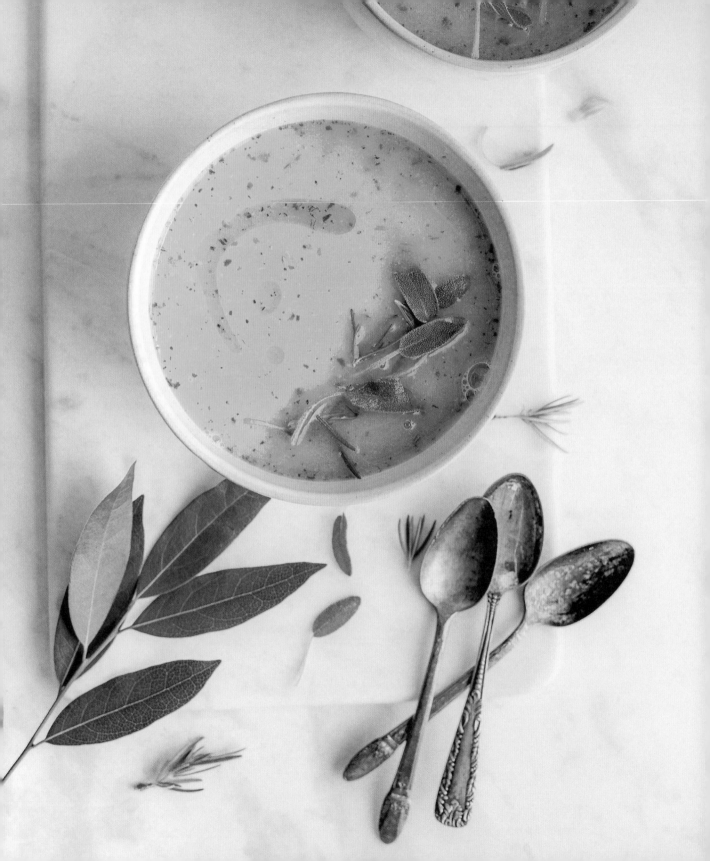

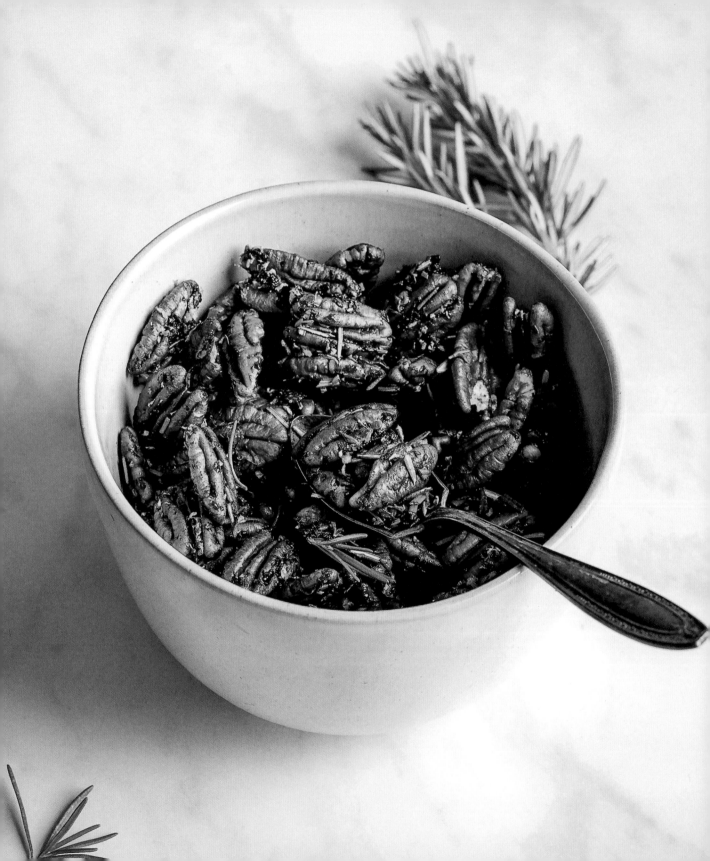

maple-rosemary pecans

MAKES ABOUT 2 CUPS

2 tablespoons Three-Herb Ghee (page 64) or unsalted butter

2 tablespoons maple sugar

½ teaspoon fine sea salt

¼ teaspoon cayenne pepper

2 cups raw pecans

3 tablespoons finely chopped fresh rosemary

2 teaspoons finely grated lemon peel

Make these pecans on the weekend and then enjoy them as an easy snack all week long. Rosemary and grated lemon peel add a pleasant, aromatic finish, and the cayenne gives the nuts a satisfying blast of heat. You can add more, of course, if you enjoy hot foods, or omit it entirely if you don't. I like to use maple sugar in this recipe for its rich, woodsy sweetness, but you can substitute coconut sugar or whole, unrefined cane sugar, too.

Preheat the oven to 375°F and line a rimmed baking sheet with parchment paper.

In a 10-inch skillet over medium heat, melt the ghee, then stir in the maple sugar, salt, and cayenne. Stir in the pecans with a spatula and then transfer to the prepared baking sheet.

Arrange the pecans in a single layer and bake them for about 10 minutes, stirring occasionally.

Transfer the pecans to a bowl, stir in the rosemary and lemon peel, and then let cool completely before serving. You can store the pecans in an airtight container at room temperature for up to 1 week.

sage

(salvia officinalis)

Sage is a symbol of wisdom, and its unmistakable piney aroma lingers on your fingers long after you've chopped its soft, silvery-green leaves. Its Latin name, *salvia,* means "healing plant," and it is, indeed, a remarkably diverse healing plant with many and varied uses.

Herbalists value its bitterness as a digestive aid and also use the plant to help lessen symptoms of colds and sore throats. More than soothing indigestion or easing colds, sage promises to support mental clarity, quicken the senses, and improve focus. In European folk medicine, practitioners used sage to improve concentration and memory, especially in times of fatigue or stress.

Clinical research has expanded on these traditional folk uses and found that sage extracts improve cognition and memory. Similarly, compounds found in the herb protect and support brain and neuron health, especially when compromised by stress. Researchers also found sage improves alertness and concentration and can lift the mood, invoking a sense of serene contentedness.

Like most aromatic herbs, sage tastes best when you use the fresh herb. Its poignant flavor and fragrant, herbaceous perfume work well with roasted meats, earthy root vegetables, and bright citrus fruits. You can find both fresh as well as dried sage, also called rubbed sage, in most grocery stores. For medicinal use, you'll find sage in capsules and tinctures, and you can also use it in teas and herbal infusions.

Using it in the kitchen: Add fresh sage to the soup pot or blend it into bean and vegetable purees. Muddle sage with fruit and honey to make tonics and elixirs. Rubbed sage has a light, fluffy texture, and when you combine it with other dried herbs and spices, it makes a delicious rub that pairs well with poultry and meat. It also makes a soothing tisane that's especially medicinal if you have a sore throat.

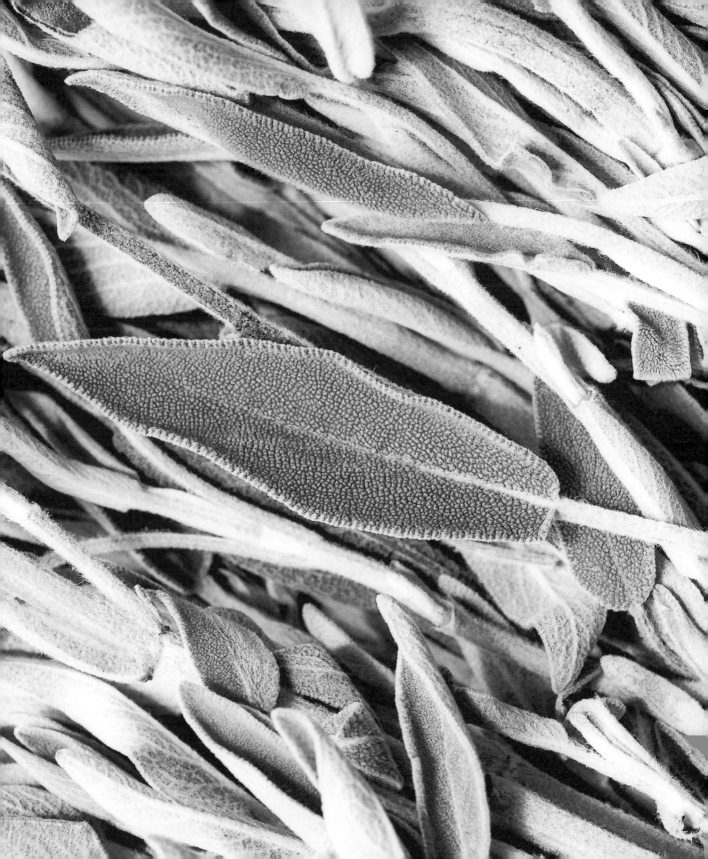

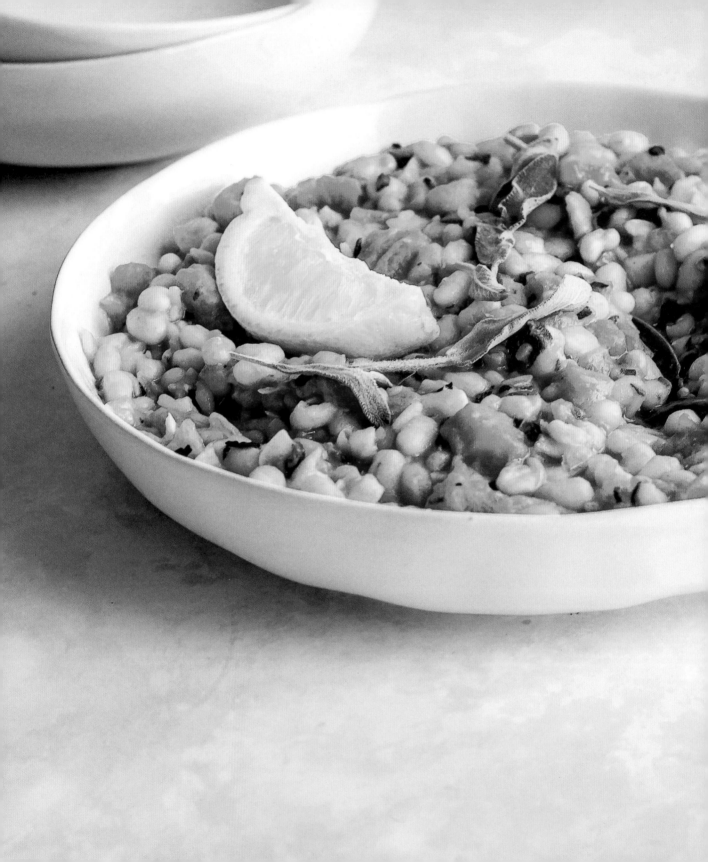

garlicky white beans with sage and tomatoes

1¼ cups small white beans, such as navy beans

1 tablespoon fine sea salt

¼ teaspoon baking soda

1 medium yellow onion, halved

1 (6-inch) strip kombu (optional)

¼ cup Rosemary and Sage Oil (page 67) or extra-virgin olive oil

8 garlic cloves, thinly sliced

½ cup chopped fresh sage

¼ teaspoon crushed red pepper flakes

1½ pounds fresh plum tomatoes, diced

2 lemons, quartered, for serving

I like to ladle these garlicky beans into bowls, served with slices of toasted sourdough bread and a squeeze of lemon. Garlic (see page 92) mellows with cooking, and the sage perfumes the beans with its green, piney aroma. Kombu, a seaweed used in traditional Japanese cookery, adds minerals to this dish and contains an enzyme that makes the complex starches in beans easier to digest without impacting flavor.

Sage has a remarkable effect on building and supporting cognitive health, and it partners well with olive oil and tomatoes.

Place the beans in a medium mixing bowl and pour in enough hot water to cover by 2 inches. Stir in the salt and baking soda and let the beans soak for at least 8 and up to 24 hours. Drain through a colander and rinse the beans thoroughly.

Transfer the beans to a Dutch oven or stockpot and pour in enough water to cover by 3 inches. Toss in the onion and kombu (if using) and bring the beans to a boil over medium-high heat. Immediately turn the heat down to medium-low and simmer the beans until tender, about 45 minutes.

Turn off the heat, and then ladle ½ cup of the cooking liquid into a bowl or jar and set it aside. Drain the beans in a colander and discard the onion and kombu.

In a braising dish or wide skillet over medium heat, heat the oil. Toss in the garlic, sage, and red pepper flakes, frying them together until fragrant, about 3 minutes. Stir in the plum tomatoes, coating them with oil and allowing their juices to turn syrupy, about 8 minutes more.

Spoon the beans and reserved cooking broth into the tomatoes, stirring well. Simmer for about 10 minutes, and then serve hot with a squeeze of lemon.

Leftovers will keep, in an airtight container, in the refrigerator for up to 5 days or in the freezer for up to 8 months.

blackberry sage limeade

MAKES ABOUT 2 CUPS (ENOUGH FOR 8 SERVINGS)

1 cup freshly squeezed lime juice, from about 8 limes

¾ cup honey

12 ounces blackberries

¼ cup chopped fresh sage

1 green cardamom pod

Sparkling water for serving

This is a drink you make to share. Blackberries' sweet and tart flavor finds complement with sage's citrusy top notes, while lime and cardamom bring it all together. If you can find blackberry honey in your local farmers' market, try using it in this recipe, as the fruity and floral notes in the honey will complement the berries. While I usually stir the concentrate into an icy glass of sparkling water, you can also stir it into gin for a delicious summer cocktail.

Sage has a long history of use as a nootropic, or an herb that supports memory and concentration. Its very name is a synonym for wisdom. While sage's benefits for brain health are well recognized historically as well as in the contemporary herbal community, the benefits of blackberry are less well-known but still quite promising. The volatile oils in sage and the antioxidants in blackberries help protect cells and the brain against oxidative damage and promote better memory performance.

In a small saucepan set over medium heat, whisk together the lime juice and honey until the honey dissolves. Turn off the heat, and then toss in the fresh blackberries, sage, and cardamom pod. Mash them together in the lime-honey syrup using a potato masher or the back of a wooden spoon. Let them steep until the mixture cools to room temperature, about 30 minutes.

Transfer the contents of the saucepan to a blender and puree until uniformly smooth. Strain the blackberry-sage mixture through a fine-mesh sieve into a quart-sized Mason jar, discarding the solids. Seal, label, and transfer the jar to the refrigerator, where the syrup will keep for about 1 week.

To make the limeade, fill a glass halfway with ice cubes and then pour in about ¼ cup of the syrup. Next, pour in enough sparkling water to fill the glass, stir, and serve immediately.

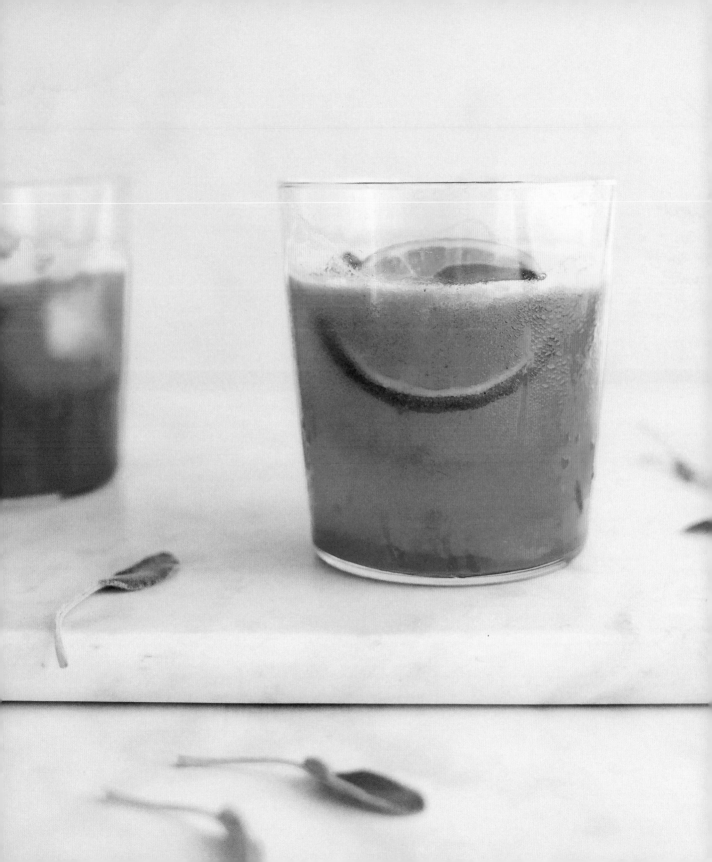

saffron
(crocus sativus)

The saffron crocus blooms in autumn, opening its delicate and elongated purple flowers to reveal three threadlike crimson stigmas. Harvesters tenderly pluck these long red threads from the blossoms by hand and then dry them. While the crocus grows readily in full sun, even in rocky soil, the labor-intensive process of harvesting the stigmas makes saffron one of the most expensive spices in the world. It's also one of the loveliest to use in your kitchen, with a subtle honeylike sweetness and faint pungent flavor. The red threads give anything you cook a deep gold-orange color, too. That potent color heralds the presence of antioxidant pigments that bestow the herb with its medicinal qualities.

Crocin is one of the health-boosting pigments that give the herb its vivid color. These compounds are highly anti-inflammatory and are potent antioxidants. Crocin is a neuroprotective compound, meaning that it helps support and protect the brain and nervous system. Accordingly, some herbalists use saffron in combination with other herbs to support brain health, concentration, and memory.

Due to its rarity and expense, saffron is sometimes adulterated and mislabeled. Yellow safflower petals turn an orangey-red when dried and bear a passing resemblance to true saffron threads. Unscrupulous sellers sometimes market safflower as saffron to unwitting spice hunters. With a keen eye, you can tell the difference between them. True saffron threads are crimson red, relatively elongated, and very thin, but the imposter safflower looks orange in color and is short and stubby. It's often marketed at an unbelievably low price, too. Likewise, avoid powdered saffron, which is also often adulterated by safflower or calendula.

As with other herbs, saffron's labor-intensive harvest leaves workers open to exploitation, so make your purchases mindfully, looking for fair trade options or purchase from companies with transparent practices.

Using it in the kitchen: Soak saffron threads in a bit of water before using them to release their pigments. Saffron's flavor complements seafood, whole grains, vanilla, and rose. Saffron tinctures are a popular remedy for anxiety.

slow-roasted saffron chicken with rosemary

MAKES 6 SERVINGS

1 whole chicken
(about 3½ pounds)

1 lemon, halved crosswise

½ teaspoon whole black peppercorns

1 teaspoon saffron threads

1 tablespoon fine sea salt

2 tablespoons extra-virgin olive oil

2 garlic cloves, finely chopped

1 cup chicken bone broth

2 tablespoons unsalted butter

2 teaspoons finely chopped fresh rosemary

Cooking poultry at low, slow temperature ensures marvelously tender meat and crisp skin. While slow roasting takes a little more time, this chicken needs very little active preparation time, which means big flavor for minimal effort. You can serve it with rice or roasted potatoes, but it also makes a great companion for the Roasted Carrots with Dukkah (page 145) and a big green salad dressed with lemon and olive oil.

Preheat the oven to 400°F.

Prick the chicken all over with a fork so that the bird releases its fat while it cooks. Stuff the bird's cavity with the lemon halves and then truss it by tucking its wings behind its back and tying its legs together.

In a spice grinder, or using a mortar and pestle, grind the black peppercorns with the saffron threads and salt and then stir the ground herbs into the olive oil.

Brush the bird all over with the olive oil and spice mixture and then transfer it to the oven. Turn down the heat to 225°F and roast for about 90 minutes, until it reaches an internal temperature of 165°F and its juices run clear.

Transfer the bird to a serving platter and let it rest while you prepare the pan sauce.

Move the roasting pan with all the drippings to the stove and turn the heat to medium-high. Stir in the garlic and let it cook in the hot fat for about 3 minutes, until fragrant. Pour in the broth and bring to a simmer, taking care to scrape up any browned bits sticking to the bottom of the pan. Simmer until the liquid reduces by half, then turn off the heat and whisk in the butter and rosemary. Serve alongside the chicken.

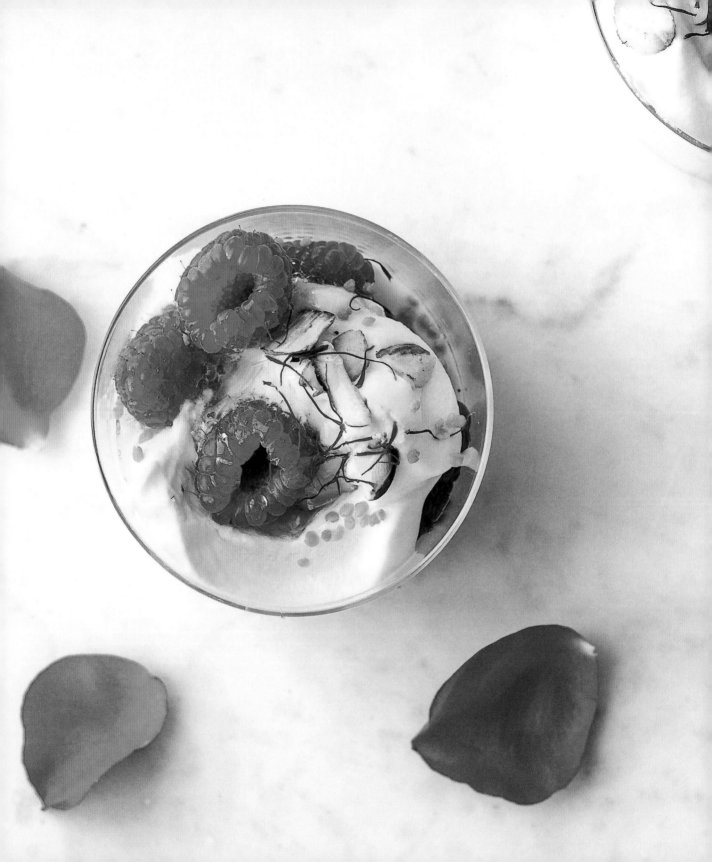

raspberries with saffron-rose cream

MAKES 4 SERVINGS

1 pinch saffron threads

2 tablespoons rose water

¾ cup heavy cream

½ cup chopped raw almonds

1 pound fresh raspberries

2 teaspoons bee pollen (optional)

Honey for drizzling

There's a cluster of raspberry canes that grow tangled among the wild briar roses outside my bedroom window. In the spring, their white blossoms attract hummingbirds who flit and buzz past the window in flurries of two or three at a time. By late summer, those flowers fade away, and the canes hang heavy with sweet, tart red berries. I almost always serve them with fresh cream as a simple dessert. Cream's neutral flavor makes a perfect avenue for other herbs, and in this recipe it partners with vivid, astringent saffron and soft, bittersweet rose for a simple, but flavor-forward dessert.

Saffron supports memory and concentration, and it has an uplifting effect on the mood, which makes it a great partner for rose. Bee pollen has a powdery, slightly sweet flavor, and it's rich in B vitamins, which can give you an energy boost.

In a small bowl or saucer, steep the saffron in the rose water for about 10 minutes.

In a separate bowl, whip the cream until it holds soft peaks. Then strain the saffron-infused rosewater into the cream and whip until just combined.

In a 10-inch skillet over medium-high heat, toast the almonds, stirring continuously, until they begin to brown and release a pleasant, toasted aroma. Turn off the heat and spoon the almonds into a small bowl.

Spoon the raspberries into four bowls. Top with a generous dollop of whipped cream, then sprinkle them with toasted almonds and bee pollen, if desired. Drizzle with honey to your liking.

turmeric

(curcuma spp.)*

Toffee-colored skin, as thin as paper, covers turmeric rhizomes. Turmeric looks like ginger, to which it's related, and when you slice into the fresh root, you'll be greeted by vivid color. The most common turmeric, golden turmeric (*Curcuma longa*), has a brilliant orange color, but there are other varieties, too, such as black turmeric (*Curcuma caesia*), which is a vibrant blue, and white turmeric (*Curcuma zedoaria*). The plant is native to South Asia, where it has a long history of use in both food and traditional botanical medicine.

Turmeric is a highly anti-inflammatory herb that supports cellular health and shows unique promise in supporting both the brain and heart. Curcumin is the best understood compound in turmeric, and it shows significant promise in calming inflammation, boosting cognitive health, and improving memory. In some studies, curcumin also improved feelings associated with anxiety and depression.

Further, turmeric's anti-inflammatory compounds also protect the liver and help improve blood sugar balance in some people. Because of its bitter and astringent flavor, curcumin also acts as a digestive aid.

You can buy fresh golden turmeric root in many health food stores and natural markets. Powdered turmeric is also available in most shops. Look for vibrant and deeply colored turmeric powders. A strong color indicates a high concentration of beneficial compounds that give turmeric both its flavor and medicinal effects. Purchase from a reputable source, as some imported turmeric powders are adulterated with lead chromate to enhance its color.

Using it in the kitchen: Peel away fresh turmeric's papery skin as you would for ginger and finely grate the root to add seasoning to stir-fries, curries, and roasted vegetables. You can also mix turmeric powder into drinks and spice blends. Turmeric's pigments are tenacious and easily stain your fingertips, countertops, and kitchen cloths, so be careful when working with the herb to prevent unwanted stains.

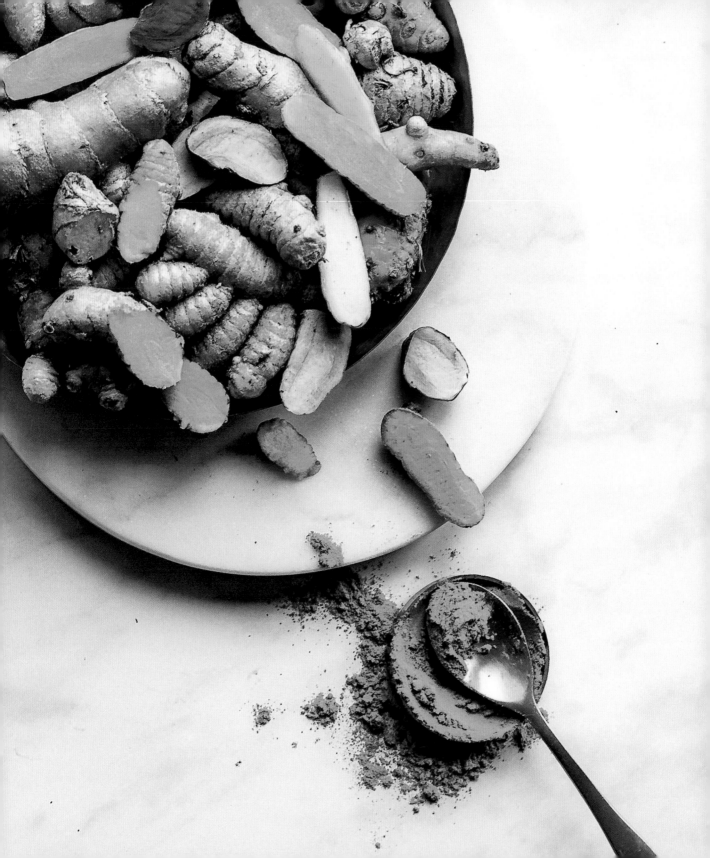

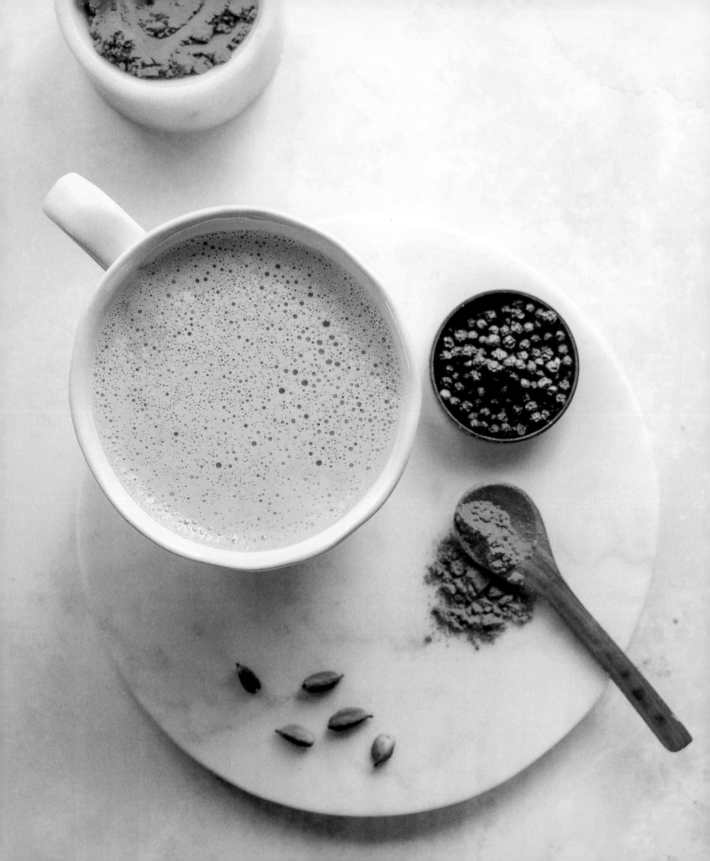

honeyed turmeric-cardamom milk

MAKES 2 SERVINGS

2½ cups whole milk

1 tablespoon turmeric powder

1 teaspoon black peppercorns

4 green cardamom pods, cracked

Honey for serving

Turmeric milk, or haldi doodh, is a traditional Indian folk remedy that's rooted in Ayurvedic medicine. In Ayurvedic traditions, turmeric helps support lung health and immune system function, so turmeric milk is often made as a comforting immune booster when you feel under the weather. Because it's such a powerful anti-inflammatory, it also supports cognitive function. Keep in mind that turmeric's medicinal compounds are best absorbed when combined with fat, which makes the traditional remedy—turmeric blended with full-fat cow's milk—particularly nourishing.

In my version, I like to add a touch of cardamom and black pepper to the turmeric and sweeten the drink with a spoonful of honey. It tastes wonderfully creamy, and its light sweetness brings balance to turmeric's natural astringency. Black pepper also has a synergizing effect on turmeric, amplifying and enhancing its benefits. If you're sensitive to dairy, you can make this drink with a blend of coconut or almond milk.

In a small saucepan over medium heat, warm the milk until it begins to steam and then whisk in the turmeric until it dissolves. Stir in the black peppercorns and cardamom pods. Turn the heat to medium-low and let the herbs warm in the hot milk for about 10 minutes, stirring occasionally.

Strain the milk through a fine-mesh sieve into two mugs and sweeten to your liking with honey. Serve hot.

turmeric turkey meatballs with cilantro-chile sauce

meatballs

1½ pounds ground turkey

2 shallots, finely chopped

1 garlic clove, finely chopped

2 tablespoons turmeric

1 tablespoon finely grated ginger

2 teaspoons fine sea salt

½ teaspoon ground coriander

½ teaspoon freshly ground black pepper

¼ teaspoon ground cumin

1 egg yolk

cilantro-chile sauce

1 bunch cilantro, including leaves and stems, coarsely chopped

1 serrano chile, seeded and coarsely chopped

2 garlic cloves, chopped

2 limes

While these turkey meatballs make an easy, nutrient-dense dinner, you can also prepare them in advance and warm them up for lunch throughout the week. Turmeric gives the meatballs a brilliant orange-gold color and a potent flavor complemented by ginger, black pepper, and coriander. Serve it with a bright sauce made from cilantro, chile, and plenty of fresh lime.

Preheat the oven to 400°F and line a rimmed baking sheet with parchment paper.

to make the meatballs: In a large mixing bowl, toss the turkey, shallots, garlic, turmeric, ginger, salt, coriander, black pepper, cumin, and egg yolk together, stirring until the ingredients are well incorporated. Working 2 tablespoons at a time, form the meat into balls about 1½ inches in diameter and set them on the baking sheet about 1 inch apart.

Transfer the meatballs to the oven and bake them for about 10 minutes, until they begin to brown at the bottom. Flip the meatballs to promote even cooking and continue baking them until well browned, about 10 minutes more.

while the meatballs cook, make the sauce: In a blender or food processor, combine the cilantro, chile, and garlic. Scrub the limes under running water, pat dry with a kitchen towel, and finely grate the lime zest over the herbs, taking care to avoid the bitter pith, and then cut the limes in half crosswise and squeeze in their juice. Process until smooth, adding water 1 teaspoon at a time, if necessary, until the sauce is blended through and about the consistency of a loose pesto.

Serve the meatballs immediately, drizzled with the sauce.

If you'd like to prepare the meatballs ahead, you can let them cool completely, then transfer them to an airtight container, where they will keep in the refrigerator for up to 5 days. When you're ready to eat, just toss them in a pan with a little broth and warm them until they're cooked through and hot. Store the sauce separately and drizzle it over the meatballs when you're ready to serve them.

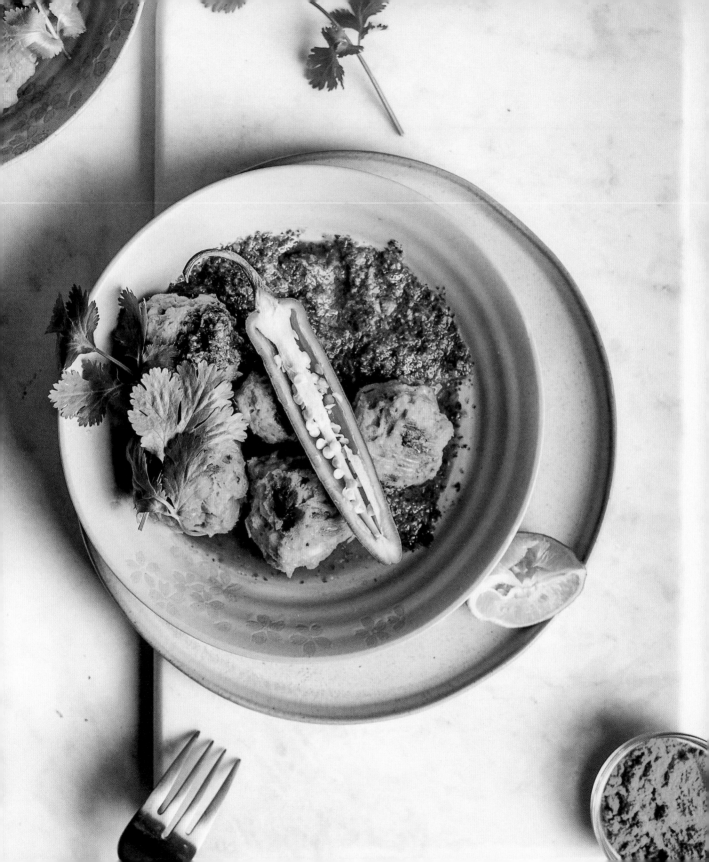

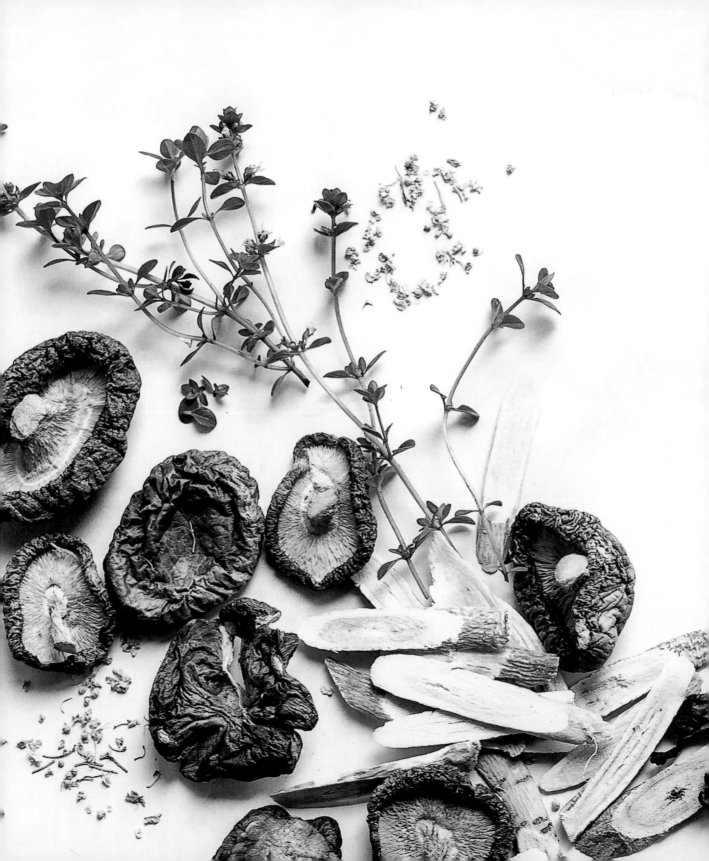

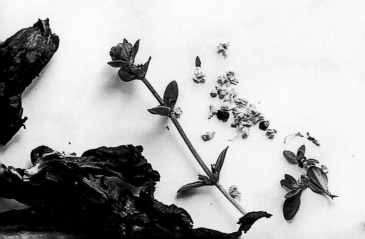

CHAPTER 4

recipes to
support immunity

When the weather takes a chill, cold and flu season arrives in a torrent of sniffles and sneezes. Since the cold and flu season approaches with some measure of rhythm and predictability, you can take early steps to support your body with gentle and effective herbal remedies that build immunity. People have long used herbs to help ward off colds, flu, and other illnesses and to shorten their duration. Gentle but effective botanical remedies can also ease symptoms when you do happen to fall sick.

Prepare yourself for colder months by regularly incorporating herbs that strengthen your immune system into your cooking. Herbs such as astragalus (see page 120) or medicinal mushrooms (see page 104) nourish your body with unique compounds that fortify the immune system, building resilience that helps your body defend itself against seasonal viruses. Immune-supportive tinctures, herbal infusions, and nourishing broths are easy to add to your weekly meal plan.

If you do find yourself sick, incorporate healing herbs into your meals. Hibiscus (see page 112) and rosehips (see page 197) are teeming with immune-supportive nutrients such as vitamin C, while garlic and other botanicals are rich in antiviral compounds. These herbs work in harmony as they strengthen your immune system, nourish your body with vital nutrients, and fight the viruses that can make you feel sick. Beyond these actions, many herbs ease symptoms directly by making coughs more productive, soothing a sore throat, or helping a fever be more effective.

herbs for immunity

Immune strengtheners: Adaptogens such as astragalus (see page 120), reishi (see page 104), schisandra berry (see page 182), and others build resilience against stress, including the stress caused by illness. They can strengthen the immune system without overwhelming it. Many medicinal mushrooms are adaptogens, and they contain special types of carbohydrates called beta-glucans that support gut health and immune system function.

Immune stimulants: Unlike adaptogens, which strengthen and regulate the immune system, other herbs, such as echinacea and elder (page 117), stimulate it. These herbs provide targeted support during cold and flu season, when you're traveling by air, or if you've been exposed to people who have been sick.

Virus busters: Antiviral herbs, such as garlic (see page 92), onion, star anise, sage (see page 72), and thyme (see page 99), support your body's efforts to fight off viruses. Many of these herbs work on a cellular level to help prevent viruses from adhering to cell walls. Emphasize them in your cooking throughout cold and flu season, or use more concentrated doses when you feel sick.

Symptom soothers: Expectorants are herbs that encourage productive coughing, and they include thyme (see page 99), oregano, sage (see page 72), and cinnamon, among others. Diaphoretics encourage sweating and may help fevers be more effective, helping your body become less hospitable to the microbes that cause illness. They include elderflower (see page 117), basil, and angelica. Analgesics, such as elder (see page 117), echinacea, mint (see page 146), and yarrow, combat inflammation and pain.

garlic
(allium sativum)

_____

Garlic grows in fat round bulbs that lead upward from the soil to a sturdy stem and elongated, pointed leaves. In the spring, garlic produces a narrow, serpentine flower called a scape. Growers cut the scape, which forces the plant to send its energy downward, growing a bigger bulb with larger cloves. Both the scape and the bulb are edible and give meals an intoxicating, delicious flavor that ranges from sharp and pungent to sweet and mellow, depending on how long you cook them.

Beyond the flavor it gives to your meals, garlic is a powerful anti-inflammatory herb. The same compounds that give garlic its intensely aromatic quality also give the plant its medicinal properties, too. They dilate the blood vessels and improve circulation, making garlic an excellent herb for heart health.

Traditionally, herbalists used garlic as a folk remedy for the common cold, especially in its early stages. Its active antiviral properties and warming energy give you comfort when you start to sniffle or feel the gnawing creep of a cold coming on. Garlic's potent volatile oils, those that give it such a pronounced odor, are also antimicrobial and make garlic a particularly good choice for upper respiratory infections. As you chew garlic, you breathe in all those potent antivirals, too.

Garlic contains sulfurous compounds that become more potent when you expose them to oxygen. So chopping or slicing garlic and letting it rest on your cutting board for a few minutes before cooking enhances the plant's medicinal properties.

You can find fresh and dried powdered garlic in any grocery store. Both offer medicinal benefits, but fresh garlic superior for cooking, lending a rounder flavor to the foods you make with it. Look for garlic flowers, or scapes, at farmers' markets and specialty grocers in the spring. Cook with the scape just as you would garlic cloves and enjoy its milder flavor.

Using it in the kitchen: Raw garlic bites the tongue with a fiery edge. Use it to bring life to vinaigrettes, salad dressings, and pestos. Cooking garlic mellows its fire, softening its flavor into a lovely savory sweetness. Sauté it with olive oil or butter, of course. Or nestle the cloves in a roasting pan alongside chicken or root vegetables.

roasted garlic and onion bisque with sage and thyme broth

MAKES 4 SERVINGS

broth

6 cups chicken broth or vegetable stock

1 tablespoon dry eleuthero root

1 bay leaf

1 teaspoon black peppercorns

10 sprigs fresh thyme

2 sage leaves

soup

1 cup peeled garlic cloves (about 40)

8 medium yellow onions, sliced ¼ inch thick

2 tablespoons extra-virgin olive oil

2 tablespoons white miso paste

Fine sea salt

Soup is always called for when you're feeling under the weather. This version beams with the savory-sweet flavor of roasted onions and garlic, blended with delicate broth infused with eleuthero, thyme, and sage. Finally, a dollop of miso paste and sprinkle of fine sea salt round out the flavor of the bisque with a savory note.

All five herbs partner well together, both in flavor and in their effect upon your body. Eleuthero's immune system support (page 35) provides an excellent foundation for both onion and garlic—two potent antivirals. In European folk medicine, herbalists use sage to soothe a sore throat and thyme to ease a cough.

to make the broth: In a medium saucepan set over medium-high heat, combine the broth, eleuthero, bay leaf, and peppercorns. Bring to a boil and then immediately turn down the heat to medium-low. Toss in the thyme and sage. Keep warm while you prepare the soup.

to make the soup: Preheat the oven to 400°F and line a rimmed baking sheet with parchment paper.

Arrange the garlic and onion on the prepared baking sheet, drizzle with the olive oil, and bake for 30 to 45 minutes, until soft and deeply fragrant, flipping the garlic and onions once halfway through.

Strain the broth through a fine-mesh strainer into a pitcher or jar, discarding the solids. Wipe the saucepan clean.

Spoon the roasted garlic and onions into the saucepan and pour in the strained broth. Simmer over medium heat for about 10 minutes. Turn off the heat, stir in the miso paste, and blend with an immersion blender until smooth. Season with fine sea salt as it suits you.

Ladle into soup bowls and serve warm.

honey-fermented garlic with bird's eye chile

MAKES ABOUT 1 PINT

24 peeled garlic cloves
(from about 3 heads)

10 bird's eye chiles

2 cups honey

Savory and sweet with a tantalizing hit of heat from the bird's eye chile, honey-fermented garlic is an excellent ally when you're feeling under the weather. Pop a clove in your mouth when you feel sick or finely chop them and add to a marinade for grilled or roasted poultry. You can also take the honey by the spoonful, and it tastes delicious drizzled over sharp cheeses.

As the garlic ferments, it releases its liquid, which causes the honey to thin and turn runny. In the first few weeks you'll see it bubble, but as fermentation progresses, that activity will quiet and the garlic will begin to darken and age. While I generally use mine within about 6 months, you can keep it for years, and the flavor will grow increasingly complex.

With a gentle hand, lightly crush the garlic cloves with the blade of your knife and drop them into a 1-pint jar. Stir in the chiles and then pour in the honey, allowing at least 1 inch of headspace. Stir it all together with a chopstick so that the honey coats each clove of garlic and no air bubbles remain. Seal, label, and tuck the jar into the cupboard away from direct light and heat for at least 1 month before using.

The jar of honey-fermented garlic will last for years stored at room temperature.

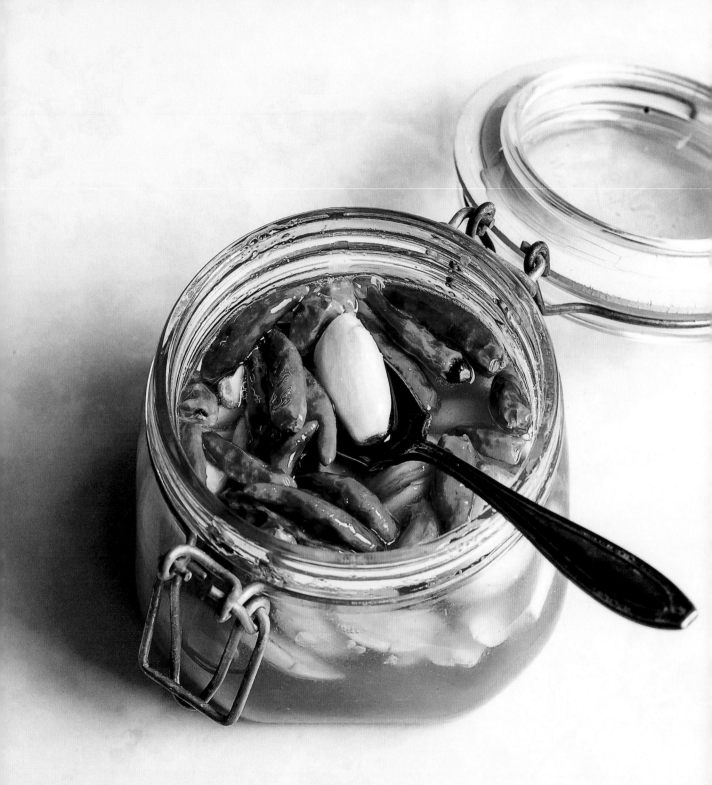

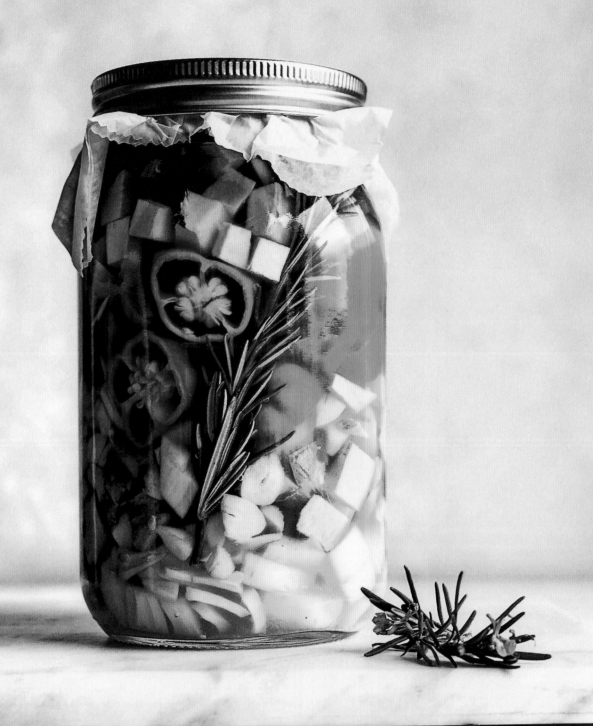

fire cider with rosemary and sage

MAKES ABOUT 2½ CUPS

1 (4-inch) knob fresh ginger, coarsely chopped

1 small yellow onion, coarsely chopped

10 medium cloves garlic, coarsely chopped

1 (3-inch) piece fresh horseradish root, coarsely chopped

6 habanero chiles, coarsely chopped

3 (4-inch) sprigs fresh rosemary

½ cup loosely packed fresh sage leaves

2 cups apple cider vinegar, plus more if needed

½ cup honey

Fire cider is a popular cold and flu remedy for the winter months. Noted American herbalist Rosemary Gladstar developed the recipe in the late 1970s, and from her work a small but passionate movement of fire cider enthusiasts was born. There are many adaptations of her original recipe, including the one that follows, which favors habanero peppers over cayenne powder and includes rosemary and sage for good measure.

Some people like to take a shot of fire cider to ward off a cold, but I prefer to use it in cooking as a base for vinaigrettes and marinades or to season steamed and roasted vegetables. It's an excellent immune boost when everyone around you seems to be coughing, sneezing, and sniffling. The heat from hot chiles and ginger (see page 128) balances the robust flavor of garlic and onion. Since fire cider is so acidic, it will corrode metal lids over time, so use a plastic or other nonmetal lid, or follow the instructions on page 21.

Place the ginger, onion, garlic, horseradish, chiles, rosemary, and sage in 1-quart jar and then pour the vinegar over them until they're completely submerged, adding more vinegar if necessary. Seal the jar, label it, and place it in your cupboard away from light and heat, shaking it daily for 1 month.

Strain the vinegar through a fine-mesh sieve into a 1-quart jar, discarding the solids, and stir in the honey. Seal the jar, label it, and store the fire cider in a cupboard away from direct light and heat for up to 1 year.

fire cider–roasted chicken breasts

MAKES 4 SERVINGS

4 split (bone-in, skin-on)
chicken breasts

1 (1-inch) knob ginger,
finely grated

2 shallots, coarsely chopped

1 tablespoon finely grated fresh
horseradish

½ teaspoon cayenne pepper

1 tablespoon fine sea salt

½ cup Fire Cider with Rosemary
and Sage (page 97) or apple
cider vinegar

½ cup extra-virgin olive oil

2 tablespoons honey

6 garlic cloves, minced

2 tablespoons minced
fresh rosemary

I love the flavors of fire cider—the heat of ginger and hot chiles, the garlic, and the bracing acidity of apple cider vinegar mellowed by just the right amount of honey. It makes an excellent marinade for chicken. Blending fire cider with plenty of extra ginger, shallots, horseradish, and cayenne gives it an even more potent flavor. Then, just before roasting, you can brush the chicken breasts with honey, garlic, and rosemary for a lovely finish. If you prefer dark meat, you can substitute chicken thighs for the breasts.

In a shallow glass dish with a tight-fitting lid or a resealable, food-safe plastic bag, arrange the chicken in a single layer.

In a blender, combine the ginger, shallots, horseradish, cayenne, salt, fire cider, and olive oil. Blend until smooth. Pour the marinade over the chicken, seal, and let marinate for at least 2 hours and up to overnight.

Preheat the oven to 400°F and line a rimmed baking sheet with parchment paper.

Remove the chicken from the marinade, pat it dry with a kitchen towel, and then arrange it on the prepared baking sheet. Drizzle the chicken with honey, sprinkle with garlic and rosemary, and bake for 25 minutes, until it reaches an internal temperature of 165°F. Let the breasts cool for about 10 minutes and then serve.

thyme

(thymus vulgaris)

Thyme is a small plant in the mint family with thin, wiry stems and fragrant little round leaves. Its pale purple flowers open in the spring and summer, providing food for bees and other pollinators. An aromatic plant with a pleasant taste, thyme is beloved for its culinary uses, but it's also an excellent herb to combat inflammation and ease coughs and colds.

In Europe, herbalists use thyme syrups and tisanes to soothe coughing fits and bronchitis. Similarly, traditional Chinese medicine associates the herb with the lungs, and it's thought that thyme helps disperse cold energy and loosen phlegm. While current research on thyme's beneficial effects is relatively scarce, one German study found that thyme helped lessen the duration of coughing fits in people with bronchitis by 2 days.

Like many herbs in the mint family, thyme is also a relaxing herb, thought to ease anxiety and support restful sleep. When you're fighting a cold or have a nagging cough that keeps you up at night, thyme's combined effects can be an asset, as it both soothes a cough and calms the nerves.

Using it in the kitchen: As a popular culinary herb, you can find both fresh and dried thyme throughout the year in most supermarkets. The fresh plant, rich in volatile oils, tends to be more fragrant and robust in flavor than the dried herb. Use thyme in infusions and teas or drop a few sprigs into a hot, nourishing broth for a boost of flavor.

garlic and thyme oxymel

1 cup garlic cloves, chopped

¼ cup chopped fresh thyme

¼ cup chopped fresh sage

1 cup apple cider vinegar, plus more if necessary

½ cup honey

Honey-rich oxymels are an ancient remedy with roots in Greece and Persia. Its name translates to "acid and honey," and the beautiful sweet-sour blend of vinegar and honey makes oxymels a pleasant way to incorporate bitter and strong-tasting herbs in your botanical medicine cabinet. The sweet taste of honey can disguise or, at the very least, balance bitter herbs, softening the flavor and increasing their palatability.

If you have a nasty cough or a sore throat, you can take this oxymel straight off the spoon as a fast remedy, but I like to use oxymel as a replacement for vinegar in vinaigrettes and salad dressings. The blend of garlic and herbs makes it an excellent match for most salads, and all you need to do is whisk the oxymel into a little mustard and olive oil.

Spoon the garlic, thyme, and sage into a 1-pint jar and cover with the vinegar. Add more vinegar to cover the herbs, if necessary. Seal the jar (see page 21 on how to avoid corrosion), label it, and then set it in a dark cupboard for 4 to 6 weeks, shaking the jar daily.

Strain the vinegar through a fine-mesh sieve into a small saucepan and discard the solids. Warm the herb vinegar over low heat, swirl in the honey, and stir until fully dissolved.

Transfer the oxymel to a clean jar, seal, label, and store in the refrigerator for up to 6 months.

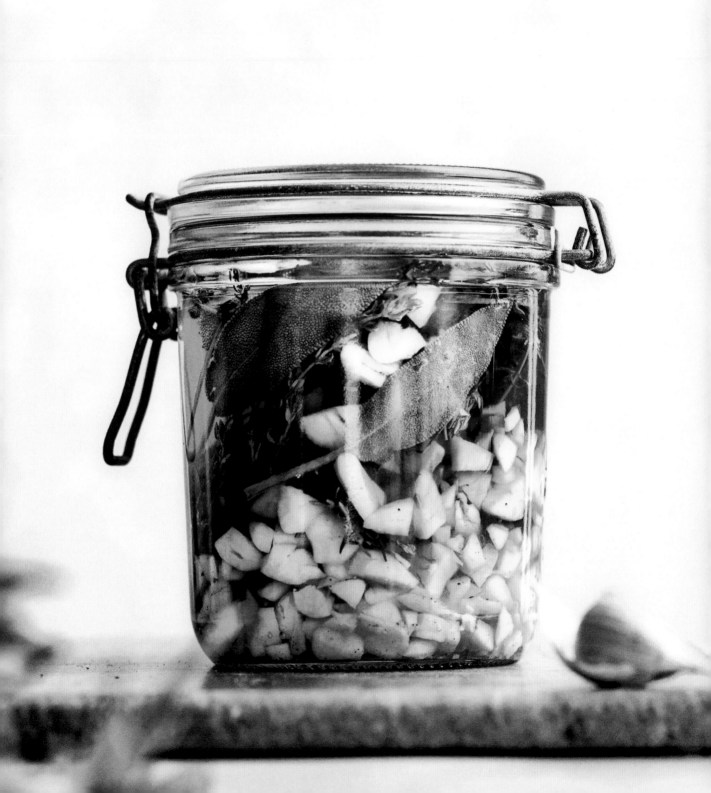

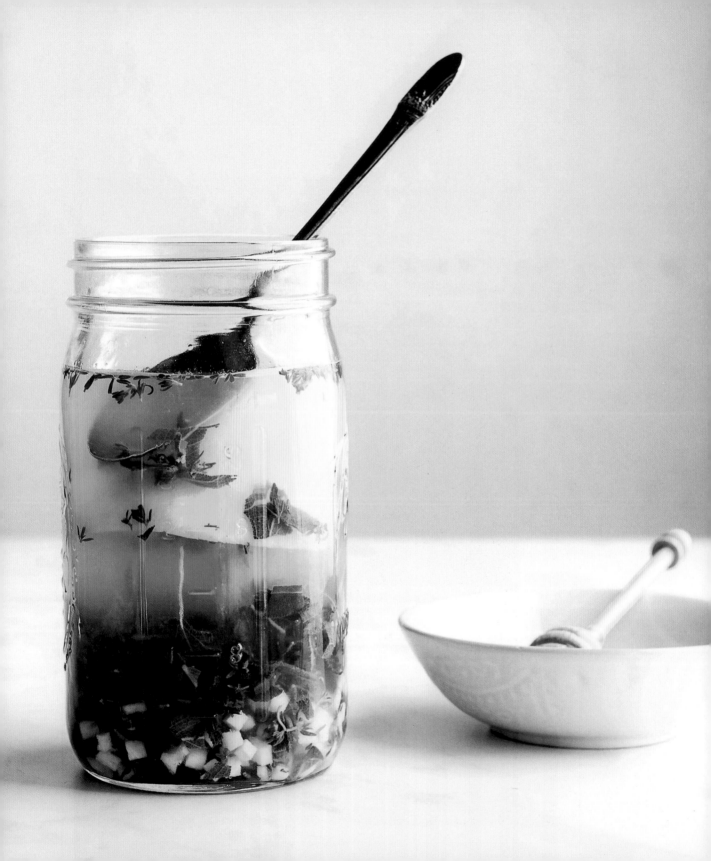

thyme and sage tisane

MAKES 2 SERVINGS

2 tablespoons chopped fresh thyme

2 tablespoons chopped fresh sage

1 (2-inch) knob ginger, coarsely chopped

1 lemon, halved crosswise

3 cups boiling water

Honey for serving

In addition to supporting cognitive health and memory, sage is also a potent antimicrobial herb. Thyme and sage tisane, with its fragrant aroma and astringent taste, can soothe a sore throat. Vibrant lemon and fiery ginger make it all the better, too, complementing sage's antiviral effects. You can add honey, if you like, to sweeten it, or drink it plain. Thyme and sage infusions, like this tisane, are potent and best avoided if you're pregnant or breastfeeding.

Place the thyme, sage, and ginger in a 1-quart jar and then squeeze in the lemon halves before plopping them in the jar as well. Pour the boiling water over the herbs, cover the jar, and let the herbs steep for about 10 minutes.

Strain the tisane through a fine-mesh sieve into two mugs and serve immediately.

medicinal mushrooms

All mushrooms, even the common button mushroom, are richly nutritious and hold a healing power deep within their cells. They tend to be a good source of various B vitamins as well as minerals such as phosphorus, potassium, and copper. Further, when exposed to sunlight, they can manufacture trace amounts of vitamin D, a vital nutrient for immune and reproductive health. They also contain a distinct and healing form of carbohydrate called beta-glucans that helps nourish gut health while building and strengthening immunity.

You can harvest mushrooms from the wild in the spring and autumn. Since some mushrooms are toxic, always hunt mushrooms with a guide who is expertly familiar with regional varieties. In many upscale grocery stores and natural markets, you can find not only button but also wild mushrooms such as chanterelles, hen of the woods, and boletes. Lastly, purchase only dried medicinal mushrooms, in whole or in powdered form, from reputable sources and herb shops.

Using it in the kitchen: Cooking mushrooms, both wild and domestic, enhances their medicinal compounds while also improving your body's ability to absorb their micronutrients. Many wild mushrooms must be cooked in order to render them edible, and even domestic mushrooms are best cooked, too.

reishi
(ganoderma lucidum)

Reishi grows on hardwood with a large, ruddy brown cap rimmed with a creamy yellow. Rare in the wild, expert growers cultivate most of the reishi available in the market. It has an earthy flavor with bitter notes reminiscent of cacao. You can find dried reishi mushroom sold in thin strips or as a fine powder, and if you're very lucky, you might find them at your local farmers' market in the summertime.

Like many medicinal mushrooms, reishi is an adaptogen that nourishes the adrenal glands while fortifying the spirit against external stressors. Its gentle, calming energy brings balance to anxious moods and rest to sleepless nights. Further, it supports the immune system's ability to fight infection without overstimulating it.

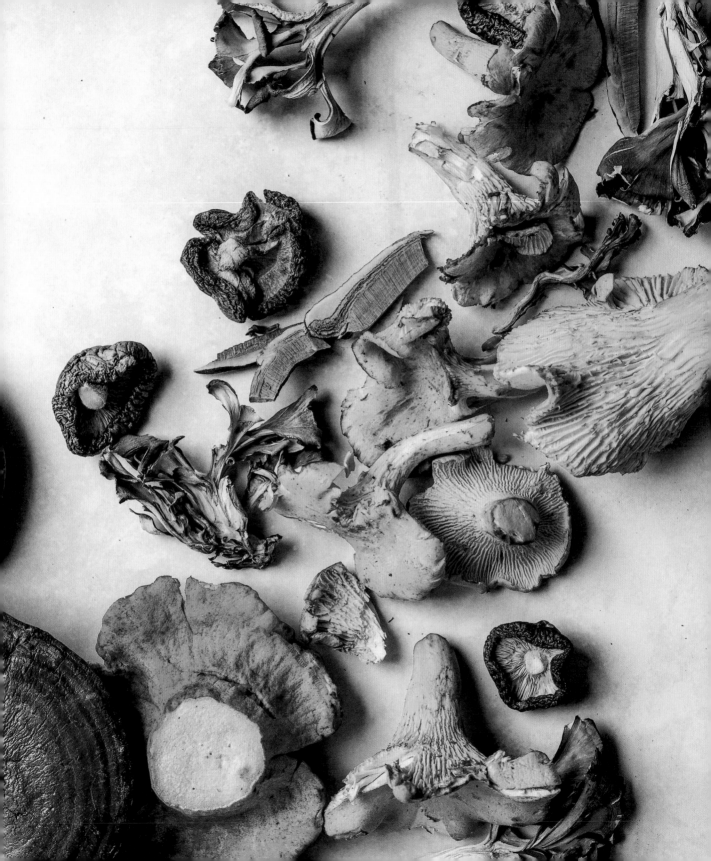

shiitake

(lentinula edodes)

Fresh shiitake mushrooms have a long stem topped by a fawn-brown cap, and you can also find them dried. They have a meaty texture and mild, sweet earthy flavor.

Shiitakes are associated with longevity, and they protect against inflammation, which is why research has mostly focused on the mushroom's ability to support heart health. They also support the liver, stimulate the immune system, and have antiviral properties.

chanterelle

(cantharellus cibarius)

The chanterelle smells faintly of apricots with a graceful hint of citrus, and it's one of the most coveted culinary mushrooms. They grow along the forest floor during the fall and winter, their golden caps nestled among spent needles and twigs beneath coniferous trees.

Chanterelles are rich in polysaccharides, or long-chain carbohydrates, that nourish the gut and support the immune system. They're also a good source of various anti-inflammatory compounds that benefit the brain and nervous system.

oyster

(pleurotus ostreatus)

Oyster mushrooms grow in spanning clumps on hardwood trees. Their creamy caps have a mild flavor and meaty texture, and they taste delicious when sautéed in garlic, herbs, and olive oil.

They're a relatively good source of minerals and are traditionally used to support the heart, protect the nervous system, and improve metabolic health.

sautéed wild mushrooms with garden herbs

1½ pounds mixed wild mushrooms, such as chanterelle, bolete, lobster, or oyster mushrooms

3 tablespoons extra-virgin olive oil

1 medium shallot, minced

2 garlic cloves, minced

½ teaspoon fine sea salt

¼ cup dry white wine, such as Pinot Grigio or Albariño

¼ cup chopped fresh flat-leaf parsley

¼ cup chopped fresh chives

2 tablespoons fresh tarragon leaves

1 tablespoon fresh thyme leaves

Autumn brings an abundance of wild mushrooms. Nourished by rich soil and cool weather, they'll pop from forested floors as soon as the rainy season starts. If you know what to look for and have luck on your side, you can head into the woods to hunt for the golden yellow caps of chanterelles peeking up from beds of spent fir needles or oyster mushrooms clinging to fallen trees. Fortunately, when the season's right, you can find them at well-stocked grocers, too.

One of the simplest ways to serve them is to toss them in a pan with olive oil, shallots, and garlic. Sauté them together until they soften and then finish them off with a little white wine and plenty of fresh garden herbs. If you can't find wild mushrooms, try a mix of cultivated mushrooms that you find at the store. Button mushrooms work just fine here, as do shiitakes. Also, you can swap chicken broth and a squeeze of lemon for the white wine if you don't feel like opening up a new bottle.

Clean the mushrooms by brushing off any dirt or debris and trimming any tough spots. Chop the mushrooms into bite-size pieces and set them in a bowl.

Warm the olive oil in a wide skillet over medium heat. When you feel the heat emanating off the pan, stir in the shallot and garlic. Let them cook in the hot oil until fragrant, about 2 minutes, and then toss in the mushrooms. Sprinkle with the salt and cook the mushrooms about 10 minutes, stirring from time to time, until they begin to soften and brown ever so slightly.

Pour in the wine and continue cooking another few minutes until the wine evaporates. Turn off the heat, stir in the parsley, chives, tarragon, and thyme and serve warm.

Store any leftovers in an airtight container in the refrigerator up to 3 days.

immunity broth

MAKES ABOUT 3 QUARTS

2 pounds chicken bones, such as wings, backs, and necks

2 yellow onions, halved

3 bulbs garlic, halved crosswise

10 slices dried astragalus root, about 3 inches long and ¹⁄₁₆-inch thick

1 (2-inch) knob fresh ginger, cubed

8 slices dried reishi mushrooms, about 4 inches long and ⅛ inch thick

10 dried shiitake mushrooms, about 1½ inches in diameter

2 tablespoons extra-virgin olive oil

4 quarts water

½ cup dry white wine

6 green onions, coarsely chopped

1 cup coarsely chopped cilantro leaves and stems

Fine sea salt

When the weather turns cold, and everyone around you starts to sniffle and sneeze, make this broth. Medicinal mushrooms and astragalus root (page 120), which support the immune system without overstimulating it, fortify the broth with a savory flavor while ginger gives it a punch of brightness. White wine gives the broth the subtlest hint of acidity, which balances the earthy notes of medicinal mushrooms and complements the brightness of green onions and cilantro.

Sip the broth on its own, dressed with chopped fresh garlic or a spoonful of finely grated ginger, or use it as the foundation of a nourishing soup filled with diced fresh vegetables and finely chopped herbs. It also freezes beautifully, and you can make it ahead and pull it out of the freezer just when everyone around you seems to be getting sick.

Preheat the oven to 300°F and line a rimmed baking sheet with parchment paper.

Arrange the chicken, onion, garlic, astragalus, ginger, and mushrooms on the baking sheet and drizzle them with the olive oil. Bake until the onions soften and become deeply fragrant, about 1 hour.

Using tongs, transfer the contents of the baking sheet to a large stockpot. Pour in the water and wine. Bring to a boil over medium-high heat and then immediately turn down the heat to medium-low. Simmer, uncovered, for about 6 hours.

Turn off the heat, drop in the green onions and cilantro, and cover the pot. Let the herbs wilt in the residual heat of the pot for about 20 minutes, and then season the broth with fine sea salt to your liking.

Strain, discarding the solids. Pour the broth into jars. Serve immediately or seal and refrigerate for up to 5 days. Alternatively, you can pour the broth into 1-quart Mason jars, allowing at least 2 inches of head space, and freeze for up to 6 months.

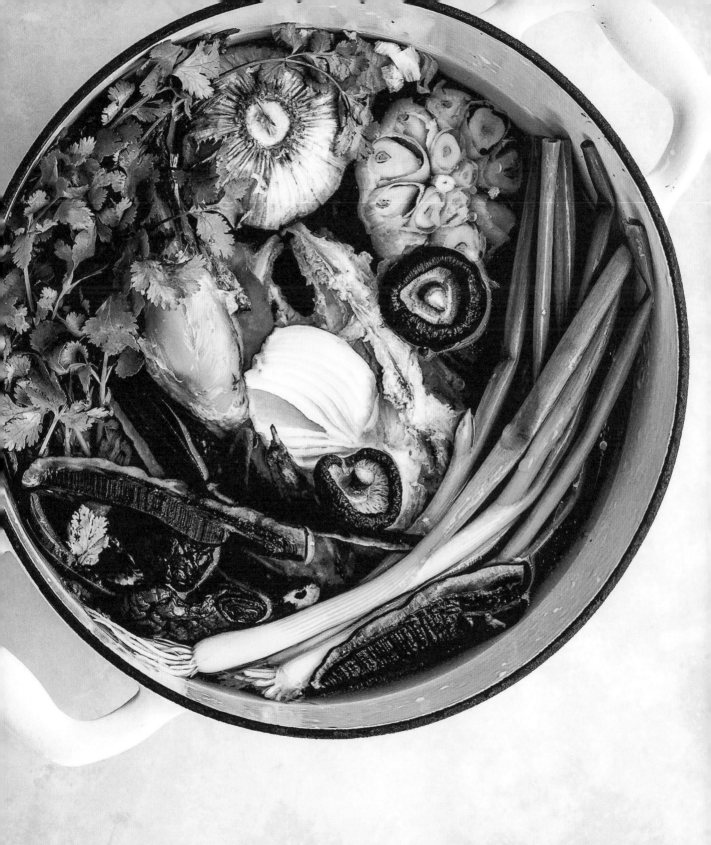

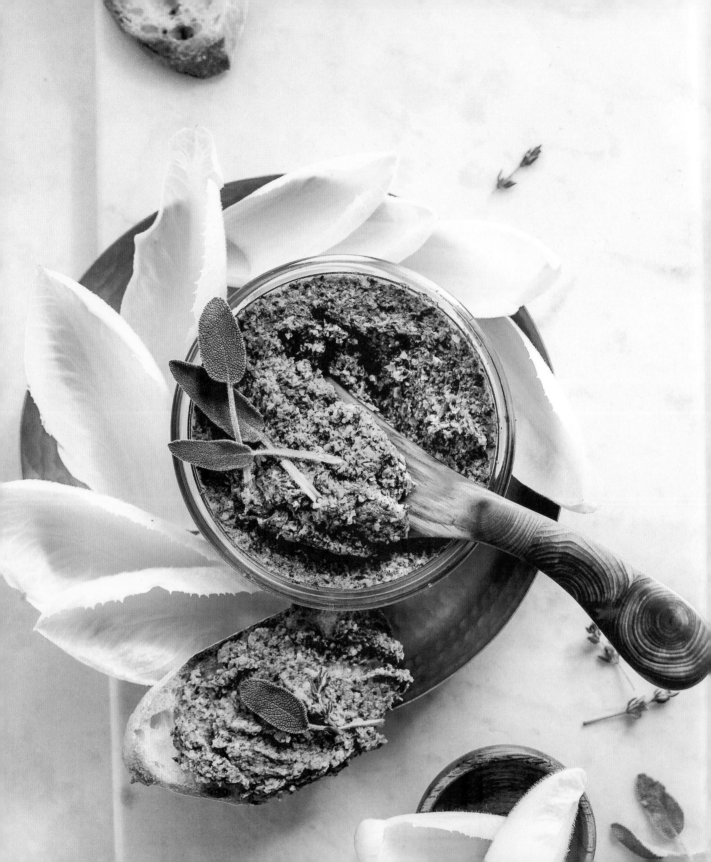

wild mushroom pâté

MAKES ABOUT 8 SERVINGS AS AN APPETIZER

1 cup raw walnuts

1 tablespoon freshly squeezed lemon juice

3 tablespoons extra-virgin olive oil

2 tablespoons salted butter

4 garlic cloves, chopped

1 medium shallot, chopped

1 tablespoon fresh thyme leaves

1 tablespoon finely chopped fresh sage

1 pound mixed fresh mushrooms, such as chanterelles, boletes, shiitake, and oyster

2 teaspoons reishi mushroom powder

¼ cup dry white wine

1 teaspoon fine sea salt

½ teaspoon freshly cracked black pepper

The trick to this pâté, or any mushroom dish, is variety. Use as many mushrooms as you can find, from the common button mushroom to wild chanterelles or hen of the woods, if you're lucky enough to stumble upon them. The greater the variety of mushrooms you use, the richer and more robust the flavor of this pâté will be. Spread the pâté on toasted sourdough bread or spoon it into leaves of Belgian endive for an easy, nourishing appetizer. Walnuts give the pâté body and creaminess, but they need to soak in advance, so make sure to start the recipe the day before you plan to serve it.

Place the walnuts in a small bowl and cover them with hot water. Squeeze in the lemon juice and allow them to soak for at least 4 and up to 12 hours, then drain and pat dry with a kitchen towel.

In a large skillet over medium heat, warm the olive oil and butter and then stir in the garlic, shallot, thyme, and sage. Sauté until fragrant, about 4 minutes. Toss in the mixed, fresh mushrooms and reishi powder and sauté for 8 minutes more, until softened. Pour the wine over the mushrooms and then scrape up any tough bits that adhere to the bottom of the pan with a spatula. Continue cooking until the liquid is mostly evaporated, about 5 minutes more.

Transfer the mushrooms to a food processor and add the soaked walnuts. Process until smooth and then spoon into a serving dish. Serve right away or cover the pâté tightly and store in the refrigerator for up to 5 days.

hibiscus

(hibiscus sabdariffa)

———

Hibiscus sabdariffa, also called roselle, blooms in large butter-yellow blossoms dotted in the center by a rich maroon. As the season wears on, the flower loses its petals and forms a plump calyx, which is something between fruit and flower. This blood-red calyx bursts with a zippy sourness and ample micronutrients.

The high concentration of vitamin C, fruit acids, and antioxidants in hibiscus give the plant both its recognizable flavor and its medicinal properties. Vitamin C and antioxidants act as potent anti-inflammatory compounds that support the immune system during times of illness. While the herb is native to Africa, it's popular throughout the world, forming the basis of refreshing drinks in the Caribbean, Mexico, and Eastern Europe, and is used to soothe sore throats and ward off the common cold. Its anti-inflammatory properties also help counteract systemic inflammation. In Iran, the herb is used as a tonic for the heart. Current research supports this traditional use, and some researchers have found that hibiscus may support heart health by lowering blood pressure and improving cholesterol levels.

Hibiscus cools inflammation. Serving hibiscus cold, in infusions or popsicles (see the opposite page), amplifies its cooling properties. You can use it fresh if you're lucky enough to find it or if you grow your own, but you're more likely to find it dried or bottled in simple syrup. I like to use the dried whole flowers, but you can also use the dried cut and sifted herbs and hibiscus powder. Look for a deep maroon color in both the whole flower and the cut herb.

Using it in the kitchen: Hibiscus is a delicate herb, so it needs a gentle touch. Tisanes and nourishing infusions (both cold and hot) work well for this herb. Use these infusions as a foundation on which you make other dishes. Hibiscus syrup, shrubs, elixirs, popsicles, and sorbets work well.

hibiscus rosehip popsicles

MAKES 10 POPSICLES

½ cup dried hibiscus flowers

¼ cup dried rosehips

4 cups boiling water

Juice of 2 limes

¼ cup honey

These sweet-tart popsicles are perfect when your throat feels a little scratchy. While the popsicle's cold temperature can make your throat feel better, it's the vitamin C packed into these that your body craves. Vitamin C gives both rosehips (page 197) and hibiscus their acidic flavor. They're also packed with various antioxidant and anti-inflammatory compounds. Both herbs strengthen the immune system and help fight off colds, and their flavors harmonize with one another, too. A swirl of honey tempers their acidity and makes for a soothing, pleasant treat.

In a 1-quart Mason jar, combine the hibiscus and rosehips, cover with the boiling water, and let steep for at least 4 and up to 8 hours.

Strain the infusion through a fine-mesh sieve, discarding the solids. Whisk in the lime juice and honey and then pour the infusion into popsicle molds. Freeze for at least 4 hours or until solid. Enjoy the popsicles within 3 months.

hibiscus pineapple punch

MAKES ABOUT 4 SERVINGS

3½ cups water

½ cup dried hibiscus flowers

2 tablespoons dried elderflower

Juice of 1 lime

2½ cups unsweetened
pineapple juice

1 cup freshly squeezed
orange juice

This hibiscus punch, brightly sour with a hint of sweetness, makes a refreshing drink in the summertime. You can dilute the punch with sparkling water or intensify it with a shot of rum if you like.

Bring the water to a boil in a medium saucepan and then turn off the heat. Stir in the hibiscus and elderflower. Cover the pot and let them steep for about 20 minutes.

Strain the liquid through a fine-mesh sieve, discarding the solids. Stir in the lime, pineapple, and orange juices and transfer it to the refrigerator where it will keep for about 3 days. Serve cold over ice.

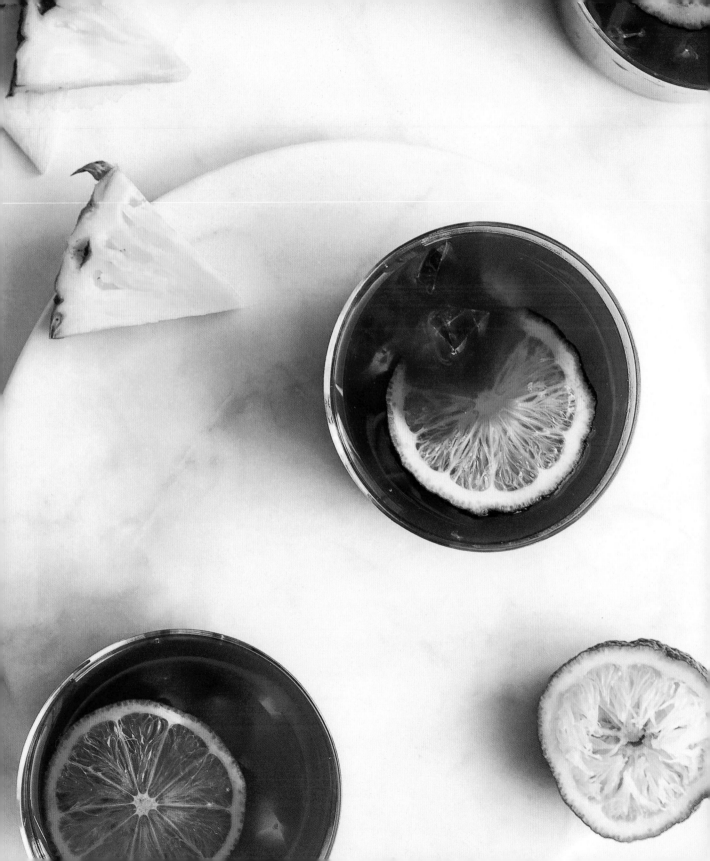

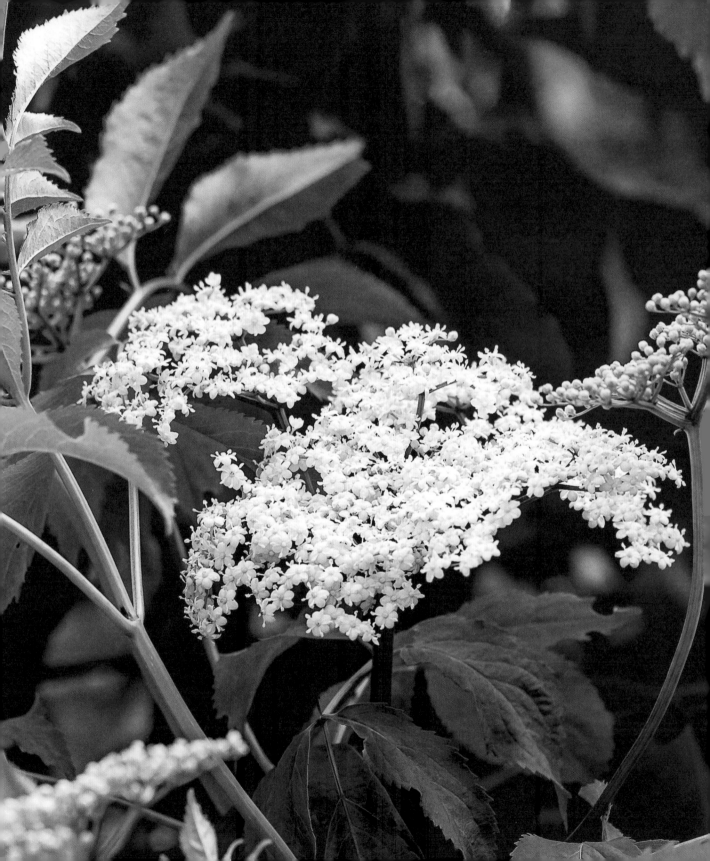

elder

(sambucus nigra)

In late spring, tiny elderflowers burst open in frilly clusters, covering the elder tree in what looks like cream-colored lace from a distance. They perfume the air around them with a musky aroma that smells very faintly of pineapple. The blossoms fade over time, growing into small plump berries the color of midnight. Both the flowers and berries have been a source of food and medicine for generations.

Elder is best known for its plump dark berry, which is a traditional folk remedy for cold and flu. It's mostly taken as a syrup, although you can serve it in tinctures, too. Rich in vitamins B_6 and C, beta-carotene, antioxidants, and other phytonutrients, elderberry supports and stimulates the immune system. Researchers studying elderberry have found that the herb lessens the severity and duration of the common cold and that it shows some efficacy against flu. It also partners well with echinacea, another herb that stimulates the immune system, as well as with ginger (see page 128), whose uplifting energy activates and harmonizes other herbs.

Like elderberry, elderflower also supports the immune system. Sipping elderflower infusions is a lovely remedy for upper respiratory tract infections. As an expectorant, elderflower clears congestion, making coughs more productive. Elderflower also soothes the nerves, and its uplifting quality can be valuable during times of stress.

You can find elderflower fresh in the spring and elderberries in early autumn. They're both available dried from specialty herb shops. Keep in mind that the uncooked fresh berries are toxic and cause indigestion, nausea, and vomiting, so always cook them thoroughly before eating them.

Using it in the kitchen: While elderberries are a popular remedy for cold and flu, they're delicious, too. You can use elderberries to make medicinal syrups that also work nicely drizzled over pancakes or swirled into sparkling water as a pleasant drink. Elderflower has a pineapple-like flavor, and it makes a lovely herbal infusion.

elderberry hibiscus jelly dessert

2 tablespoons dried elderberries

1 tablespoon dried rosehips

1 tablespoon schisandra berries

2½ cups tart cherry juice

¼ cup dried hibiscus flowers

2 tablespoons dried elderflower

1 tablespoon gelatin powder

2 tablespoons water

½ cup honey

Dark with elderberries, this simple dessert has a mild honey-like sweetness that finds balance with the pleasant tartness of rosehips and hibiscus. I make it for my children when they're feeling sick. It's a simple dessert, similar to Jello, only infused with nourishing herbal medicines. Elderberries support your body's ability to fight off viruses, while schisandra (see page 182) fortifies the immune system. Rosehips and hibiscus provide plenty of good flavor and lots of vitamin C. Tart cherry juice and elderflower (see page 117) have a calming energy that also encourages another remedy for illness: adequate rest.

In a small saucepan over medium-high heat, bring the elderberries, rosehips, schisandra berries, and tart cherry juice to a boil. Turn down the heat to medium-low, cover, and simmer for about 20 minutes, then turn off the heat.

Stir in the hibiscus and elderflower and let steep, covered, for about 10 minutes.

Meanwhile, in a small bowl, cover the gelatin with the water so that it softens.

Strain the infusion through a fine-mesh sieve into a medium bowl, discard the solids, and then whisk in the softened gelatin and the honey. If the juice is too cool to incorporate the gelatin, you may need to return it to a clean saucepan and warm it up so that the gelatin dissolves easily.

Pour the mixture into a quart-sized baking dish, cover it tightly, and transfer it to the refrigerator. Let the gelatin set for at least 8 hours, and then serve in portions of ½ cup to ¾ cup. It'll keep for about 3 days in the refrigerator.

elderberry ginger syrup

MAKES ABOUT 1 PINT

2 cups dried elderberries

¼ cup chopped fresh ginger

2 tablespoons dried rosehips

2 tablespoons dried orange peel

2 cups water

¼ cup dried elderflower

½ cup honey

Herbalists have used elderberries for ages to speed recovery from cold and flu, and elderberry syrup is, perhaps, one of the most popular remedies. Adding ginger, rosehips, and orange peel give the syrup a zip of extra flavor. While the syrup is undoubtedly filled with medicinal compounds, it's also delicious. Take it off the spoon when you feel as if you're coming down with a bug or enjoy 1 to 2 tablespoons stirred into mineral water and served over ice for a pleasant, immune-boosting tonic.

In a medium saucepan over medium-high heat, bring the elderberries, ginger, rosehips, orange peel, and water to a boil, then immediately turn down the heat to low. Simmer, uncovered, for 30 minutes.

Turn off the heat, stir in the elderflower, and let steep for 1 hour.

Strain the liquid through a fine-mesh sieve, discarding the solids. Whisk in the honey until fully dissolved and then transfer to a clean 1-pint Mason jar. Store in the refrigerator for up to 3 months.

astragalus

(astragalus propinquus)

Astragalus is a woody root that tastes faintly sweet, with subtle hints of ginger. Native to China and Mongolia, the herb has been used in traditional Chinese medicine for thousands of years and is rapidly gaining popularity owing to its stress-reducing and immune-supportive properties.

As an adaptogen, astragalus supports your body's ability to handle stress. It also strengthens the immune system by supporting the growth of white blood cells and antibodies. In clinical trials, the herb showed immune-regulating and antiviral activity. This makes it an excellent restorative herb to build resilience and promote a state of general wellness, especially in the winter months, when everyone around you is falling sick.

Beyond its ability to support your body's stress response and immune systems, astragalus supports the heart, protects liver health, and encourages better blood sugar balance. These benefits mostly come from the herb's anti-inflammatory activity and its many antioxidants and complex carbohydrates.

Astragalus is also a nourishing herb. It contains various minerals, including in selenium, a mineral that supports thyroid health and acts as a potent antioxidant. It also contains zinc, which strengthens immunity and reproductive health.

Herb shops sell dried astragalus root in thin, woody slices and as a powder. Avoid capsules when you can, as they're prone to adulteration, and always look for a supplier that uses organic methods, to reduce your exposure to synthetic pesticides and other agriculture inputs.

Using it in the kitchen: You can take astragalus as a tincture or make a nourishing herbal infusion from the root. Alternatively, drop a few slices into a simmering pot of soup or a whole-grain porridge, remembering to remove the woody root before serving. You can also fold powdered astragalus into homemade truffles, date bars, or baked goods.

echinacea and astragalus tincture

MAKES ABOUT 8 OUNCES

¼ cup cut and sifted dried echinacea root

2 tablespoons cut and sifted dried astragalus root

2 tablespoons dried schisandra berries

1 cup 100-proof distilled alcohol, such as vodka

This tincture combines echinacea with astragalus and schisandra berry, which work in concert with one another. While echinacea stimulates the immune system, a blessing when the sniffles are going around, astragalus and schisandra (page 182) help regulate it, while just a touch of ginger has a harmonic effect on the other herbs. I take a dropperful under the tongue when people around me begin to fall sick. While you can store tinctures and bitters in small pint-size Mason jars, pick up a few 8-ounce Boston round bottles as they're perfect for keeping your botanical medicines. When making tinctures, use a jar with a nonmetal lid or see page 21 for other tips on preventing corrosion.

Spoon the echinacea, astragalus, and schisandra into a 1-quart Mason jar and then cover with vodka. Seal the jar, label it, and then tuck it in dark place in your kitchen that's inaccessible to children. Shake the jar twice daily for 1 month, and then strain the liquid through a fine-mesh sieve into a clean 8-ounce bottle, discarding the solids.

Seal the jar, label it, and store it in a cupboard away from direct light and heat where children can't reach the tincture. Take a dropperful under the tongue and use the tincture within about 2 years.

spiced astragalus tea

MAKES 2 SERVINGS

10 slices dried astragalus root

1 (3-inch) knob fresh ginger, sliced thin

2 cinnamon sticks

4 green cardamom pods, cracked

3 star anise pods

2 teaspoons fennel seeds

1 teaspoon whole black peppercorns

3 cups cold water

2 teaspoons black tea, such as Assam

1 cup milk

Honey or unrefined cane sugar for sweetening

The subtle sweetness of astragalus marries beautifully with ginger and cardamom. Together, they work well in this recipe for spiced tea, reminiscent of traditional Indian chai masala with its invigorating yet soothing blend of sweet and warming spices. Cinnamon, black pepper, and fennel give the drink a rich depth while star anise adds a sweet spiciness and bolsters its antiviral properties.

Drinking the tea regularly, especially during winter months, can warm your spirit and strengthen your immune system when you need it most. The trick is to let the hardy herbs—roots, pods, and seeds—simmer long enough to release their beneficial compounds without oversteeping the tea and turning your brew unpleasantly tannic and bitter. So, prepare a decoction of the tougher herbs and toss the tea in at the very end and steep only long enough for it to release its pleasant flavor without turning bitter. Add milk and then sweeten it to your liking. Honey works well, of course, but unrefined cane sugars such as panela and jaggery give the tea a delicious mineral-like sweetness.

In a small saucepan over medium-high heat, bring the astragalus, ginger, cinnamon, cardamom, star anise, fennel, peppercorns, and water to a boil and then immediately turn the heat down to medium-low. Simmer, uncovered, for 20 minutes and then turn off the heat.

Toss in the black tea, cover, and let steep for 3 to 5 minutes.

Strain the tea through a fine-mesh sieve, discarding the solids. Stir in the milk, sweeten with honey to your liking, and serve immediately.

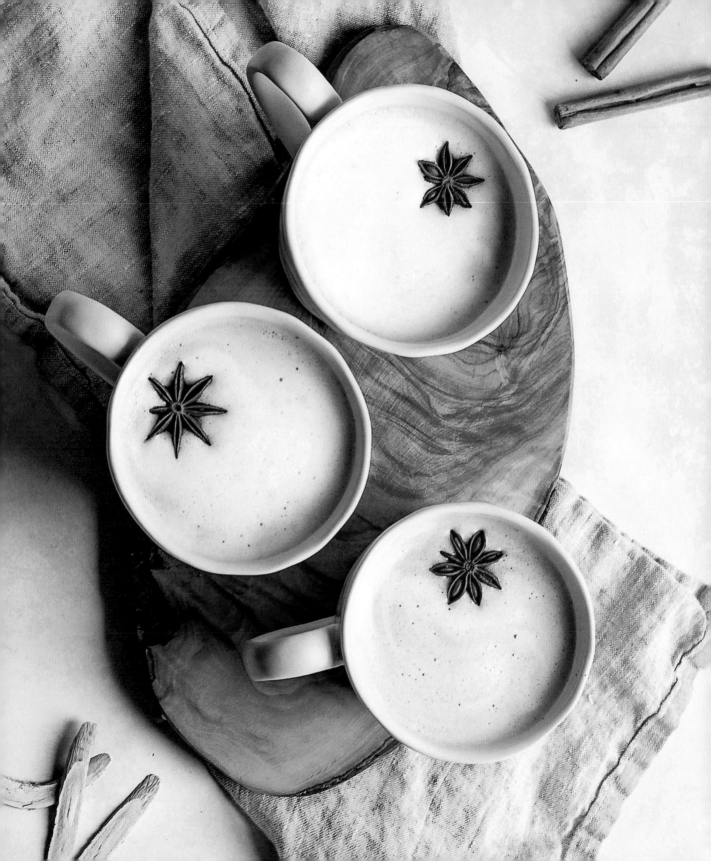

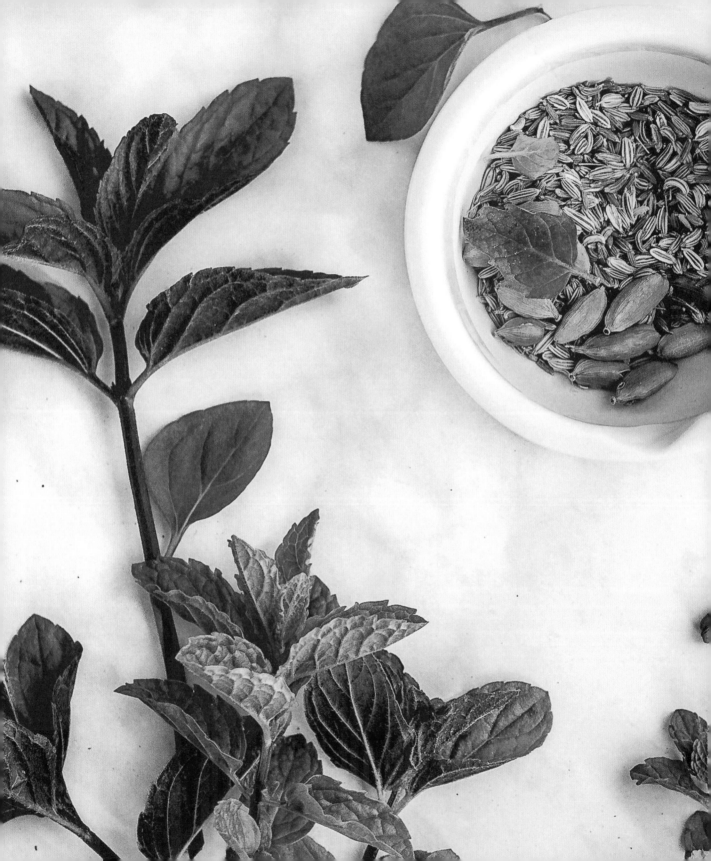

CHAPTER 5

recipes to
support digestion

Good health begins in the gut. A healthy digestive system helps your body absorb and assimilate nutrients. Digestion affects other body systems, too, including your immune system, your stress response system, and your brain. When digestion is compromised, it's difficult to absorb the nutrients you need to fuel your body or support its systemic health.

Many herbs have a natural affinity for digestion, and many culinary traditions are rooted in their use. Beginning your meal with a cocktail spiked with bitters or a salad of bitter greens dressed with lemon and olive oil helps ready your body for digestion. After-dinner mints, flavored by essential oils of spearmint and peppermint, help soothe digestion after heavy meals.

herbs for digestion

Herbs that relieve nausea: Antiemetics soothe nausea. They can be particularly helpful when stress, motion, or morning sickness upset your stomach. Ginger (see page 128), fennel (see page 141), cardamom (see page 135), and chamomile (see page 217) have stomach-soothing properties.

Bitter herbs: Bitters have an intricate relationship with the gut and nervous system. When you taste bitter flavors, your taste receptors, nervous system, and brain work together in concert and send a cascade of signals through your digestive system. These signals trigger the release of digestive juices that tell your body it's time to relax and get ready to eat. Bitter herbs include dandelion (see page 154), chicory, rosemary (see page 65), citrus peel, and chamomile (see page 217).

Herbs that tame indigestion: Deeply aromatic, carminative herbs help ease cramping, bloating, and gassiness. They often taste bittersweet with a robust, pungent flavor owing to their large concentration of volatile oils. While you can enjoy them anytime, they're particularly helpful in soothing your digestion after meals. Fennel (see page 141), cardamom (see page 135), caraway, anise, and mint (see page 146) are all carminative herbs.

Herbs to nourish a healthy gut: Prebiotics fuel probiotics, the beneficial bacteria that help support a healthy gut microbiome. Many foods and herbs contain prebiotics, and they include dandelion (see page 154), burdock, and chicory, as well as garlic (see page 92), and onion.

ginger

(zingiber officinale)

Ginger is a rhizome with a papery brown skin and a warming sweet-hot flavor. Peeling the ginger's outer skin reveals a creamy yellow vegetable that smells sharply pungent with notes of citrus and flowers. Its penetrating flavor makes it a favorite for cooking both sweet and savory foods, but it's also a powerful medicinal herb, too. To peel ginger, hold the root firmly in your non-dominant hand and a spoon in the other hand. Scrape the spoon against the root to remove its skin.

While ginger is an herb of diverse uses, its ability to ease nausea and support digestion is among its most well-known benefits. Ginger's energy is hot and fiery, and from an energetic perspective, the herb supports digestive fire. Herbalists use it to ease gassiness, bloating, and nausea. Accordingly, it's a popular remedy for morning sickness and motion sickness.

Like many of the most potent and diverse herbs, ginger owes many of its benefits to its high concentration of antioxidants and anti-inflammatory compounds. Its total antioxidant capacity is roughly three times that of blueberries. These compounds lessen inflammation, combat free radicals, and support cellular health. The anti-inflammatory effects of ginger work twofold to support systemic wellness. First, ginger helps open up the blood vessels and increases circulation, which benefits the heart and may also relieve headaches. Second, ginger promotes blood sugar balance. Together, these effects help support general wellness while combatting chronic disease.

Ginger also supports the immune system during times of illness. Researchers have found that ginger can stimulate the production of white blood cells. Further, garlic enhances that ability, and using them together is both delicious and immune-supportive.

You can find fresh ginger in any grocery store, as well as dried and powdered or candied. Fresh ginger is more potent than dried, but both are valuable, depending on how you plan to use them.

Using it in the kitchen: Sauté fresh ginger in a pan with oil to give flavor to sautéed or stir-fried vegetables or add it to the base for soups along with other aromatics such as garlic (see page 92) and onion. You can use powdered ginger in savory spice rubs or in sweet spice mixes to bring life to baked winter fruit. You can steep ginger for a few minutes in hot water to make a light tisane or, for a stronger and more medicinal brew, make a decoction to sip instead.

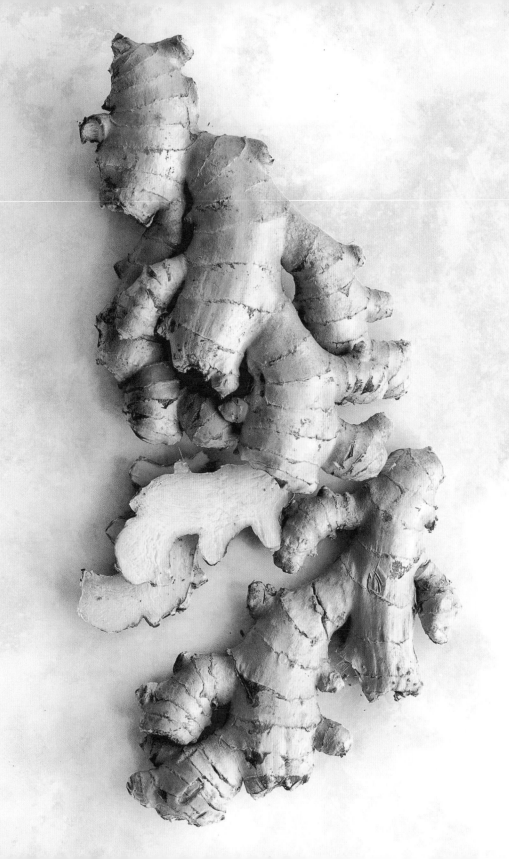

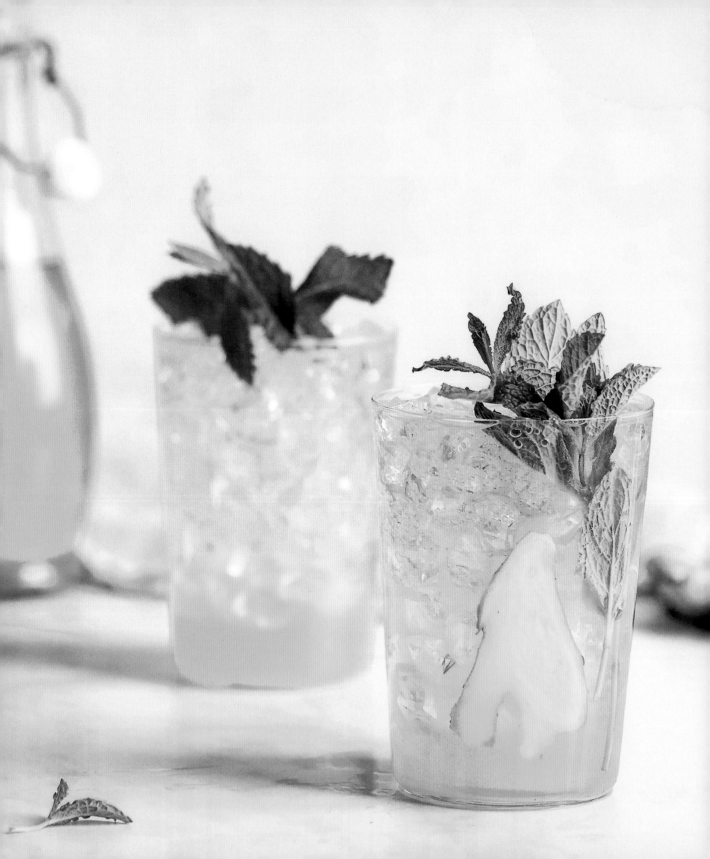

ginger mint fizz

MAKES ENOUGH FOR 12 SERVINGS

1½ cups cold water

1 (3-inch) knob fresh ginger, chopped coarsely

1 cup tightly packed chopped fresh mint

½ cup honey

Juice of 2 limes

Sparkling water for serving

Sometimes, when you're feeling a little queasy, a fizzy drink works wonders to settle your stomach. This version begins by steeping water with ginger and fresh mint to make a strong infusion. Then you swirl in enough honey to make a light syrup before adding the elixir to sparkling water. It's a delicately refreshing mix. You can serve it anytime, of course, but you might find it particularly helpful to make when you're struggling with nausea or an upset stomach.

In a small saucepan over medium-high heat, bring the water and ginger to a boil and then turn down the heat to low. Simmer, uncovered, until the liquid is reduced to 1 cup. Turn off the heat.

Stir in the mint, cover, and let steep for about 10 minutes. Strain the infusion through a fine-mesh sieve into a 1-quart Mason jar, discarding the solids. Stir in the honey and lime juice, allowing the honey to dissolve completely. Seal, label, and store the jar in the refrigerator, where it will keep for about 1 week.

To serve, fill a glass with ice, and then measure about 2 tablespoons of syrup into the glass. Cover with sparkling water and drink right away.

citus ginger bitters

MAKES ABOUT 1 CUP

1 tablespoon finely sliced orange zest

1 tablespoon finely sliced lemon zest

1 (1-inch) knob ginger, diced

8 green cardamom pods, cracked

2 teaspoons dried angelica root

1 teaspoon fennel seeds

½ teaspoon coriander seeds

8 ounces 100-proof distilled alcohol, such as vodka

Bitters add complexity and life to cocktails, but their origins are steeped in botanical medicine. Herbalists traditionally use bitters to stimulate digestion, and that's because the bitter compounds of these herbs kick-start the digestive process by encouraging the release of saliva and gastric juices. For this version, I've added angelica to a mix of citrus peel, ginger and fragrant spices. Like ginger, cardamom, and coriander, angelica has a long history of use in easing digestive discomfort. You can find it in most well-stocked herb shops and online.

Take a dropperful of these bitters under the tongue like a tincture, or stir a teaspoon into sparkling water. Both refreshing and medicinal, this remedy is particularly nice to enjoy before heavy meals.

Spoon the citrus zest, ginger, cardamom, angelica, fennel, and coriander into a 1-pint jar and then cover the herbs with the alcohol. Seal the jar (see page 21 on how to avoid corrosion), label it, and tuck it in your cupboard away from direct light and heat, shaking the jar daily for 1 month.

Strain the bitters through a fine-mesh sieve into a bottle with a tight-fitting lid, discarding the solids.

Store the bitters in the cupboard for up to 2 years.

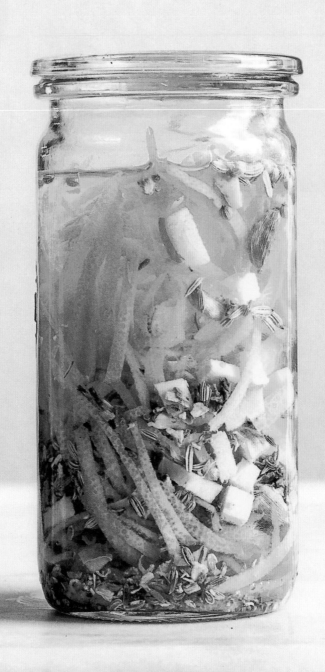

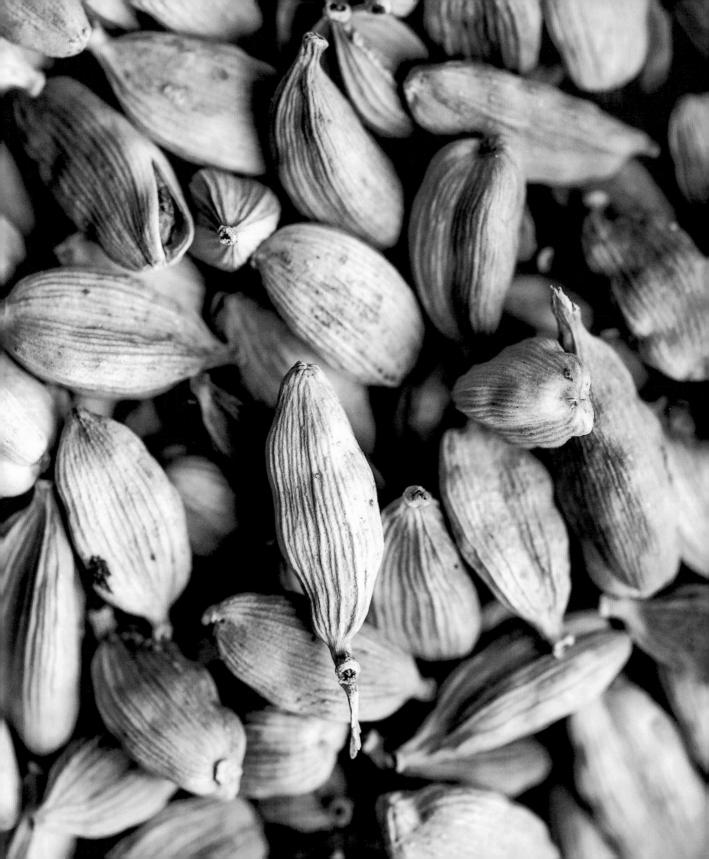

cardamom
(elettaria cardamomum)

Cardamom's pale green pods envelop a clump of dark, fragrant seeds. When you grind them, they erupt in an aromatic plume reminiscent of ginger, citrus, eucalyptus, and mint. Naturally, the spice pairs well with these herbs, and you'll find them blended together in aromatic Indian masalas and in luscious Scandinavian pastries. It's one of the most popular spices in the world and also one of the most expensive, behind saffron and vanilla.

Cardamom is a member of the ginger family. Like ginger (see page 128), it supports digestion and can ease upset stomachs. Both European folk medicine and traditional Chinese medicine prize cardamom for its ability to encourage the appetite, reduce nausea, relieve bloating, and soothe indigestion. Ayurvedic traditions also value cardamom for its ability to stimulate gastric fire and enhance digestion while also supporting liver and pancreatic health.

Volatile oils and various flavonoids give cardamom its intense aroma. They're also responsible for its medicinal qualities. Compounds such as quercetin reduce inflammation, while fragrant volatile oils increase the flow of gastric juices and bile leading to better digestion. Further, these compounds support better blood sugar balance. In a 2017 randomized controlled trial conducted in Iran, researchers found that cardamom increased insulin sensitivity and improved cholesterol levels in prediabetic women.

On an energetic level, cardamom has a hot, drying, and uplifting spirit. Its sharp, clear flavor balances bitter or earthy flavors such as coffee, tea, or chocolate. Cardamom tastes best when you grind it fresh, right before cooking. Its volatile oils are fragile, and they dissipate quickly after grinding. So, avoid the lifeless little tubs of ground cardamom in favor of the whole pod.

You can find cardamom in any well-stocked spice shop, online, and in some supermarkets. Look for whole pods with a soft green color. Old pods look dull, like green-tinged straw. Store cardamom in an airtight container, away from light to maintain its bright flavor.

Using it in the kitchen: Cardamom is assertive, and it can overpower other ingredients so use it sparingly. You can toss the whole pods into simmering liquids to bring its floral and citrus-like aroma to you herbal infusions. Ground cardamom is a common addition to fragrant curries and wintertime pastries.

spiced ghee

MAKES ABOUT 1 CUP

1 cup unsalted butter

10 green cardamom pods, cracked

2 teaspoons fennel seeds

1 cinnamon stick

Melting butter slowly and allowing its milk solids to brown, just a touch, gives ghee a toasty, nutty flavor. Cardamom, fennel, and cinnamon complement those caramel-like undertones with their sweet, spicy aroma. This spiced ghee an excellent match for the Sweet Potatoes and Apples (page 138), for homemade curries, and as a replacement for butter in spiced cakes.

In a small saucepan over medium-low heat, melt the butter, skimming off any foam with a skimmer or a spoon and discarding it. Toss in the cardamom, fennel, and cinnamon, turn the heat to low, and let the spices infuse the hot fat with their flavor for about 20 minutes, stirring occasionally.

Set a fine-mesh sieve over a 1-pint Mason jar, and then line it with cheesecloth. Strain the melted butter through the sieve into the jar. Seal, label, and store the jar at room temperature for up to 3 months or in the refrigerator for up to 1 year.

mulled cranberry cider

MAKES ABOUT 6 SERVINGS

3 cups unsweetened cranberry juice

1 cup apple cider

1 orange, cut into ¼-inch-thick slices

1 (3-inch) knob fresh ginger, coarsely chopped

2 tablespoons cardamom pods

1 tablespoon fennel seeds

1 tablespoon coriander seeds

4 star anise pods

1 cinnamon stick

Sipping mulled wine during the winter months is deliciously satisfying. The robust, tannic flavor of red wine pairs beautifully with sweet, aromatic spices. Wanting to make a version suitable for every day, I like to swap unsweetened cranberry juice for red wine and add plenty of ginger, cardamom, and other spices to make the drink positively sing. Serve it warm, in mugs, on cold nights.

In a medium saucepan over medium-high heat, combine the juice, cider, orange slices, ginger, cardamom, fennel, coriander, star anise, and cinnamon. Bring to a boil and then immediately turn down the heat to low. Simmer, covered, for about 30 minutes.

To serve, strain the juice through a fine-mesh sieve and into mugs. Or, you can strain it into a heatproof jar and set it in the refrigerator where it will keep for about 5 days. Just pour it back into a saucepan over medium heat to warm it up before serving.

sweet potatoes and apples
with fennel-cardamom dust

MAKES ABOUT 6 SERVINGS

4 medium sweet potatoes, sliced paper-thin

4 medium tart cooking apples (such as Tompkins King, Granny Smith, or Cortland), cored, halved, and sliced paper-thin

2 tablespoons melted Spiced Ghee (page 136) or unsalted butter

1 teaspoon fine sea salt

1 teaspoon ground fennel seeds

½ teaspoon ground cardamom

1 tablespoon chopped fresh thyme leaves

I like to serve this side dish in late autumn when the weather turns cold and those steadfast, nourishing root vegetables and apples find their way to the table again after a summer filled with luscious berries and robust tomatoes. Apples help balance and amplify the flavor of sweet potatoes, while digestive herbs such as cardamom and fennel seed give it a lift. Slice the apples and sweet potatoes paper-thin so they'll crisp at the edges and then cook to a melting tenderness. A mandoline is especially helpful for achieving that thinness, but a deft hand and a sharp knife work fine in a pinch.

Preheat the oven to 400°F.

In a 10-inch-round casserole dish, arrange the sweet potato and apple slices vertically in alternating layers. Drizzle the ghee over the sweet potatoes and apples, and then sprinkle them with the salt, fennel, and cardamom.

Bake for about 45 minutes, until the sweet potatoes and apples are cooked through and tender. Sprinkle with fresh thyme and serve hot.

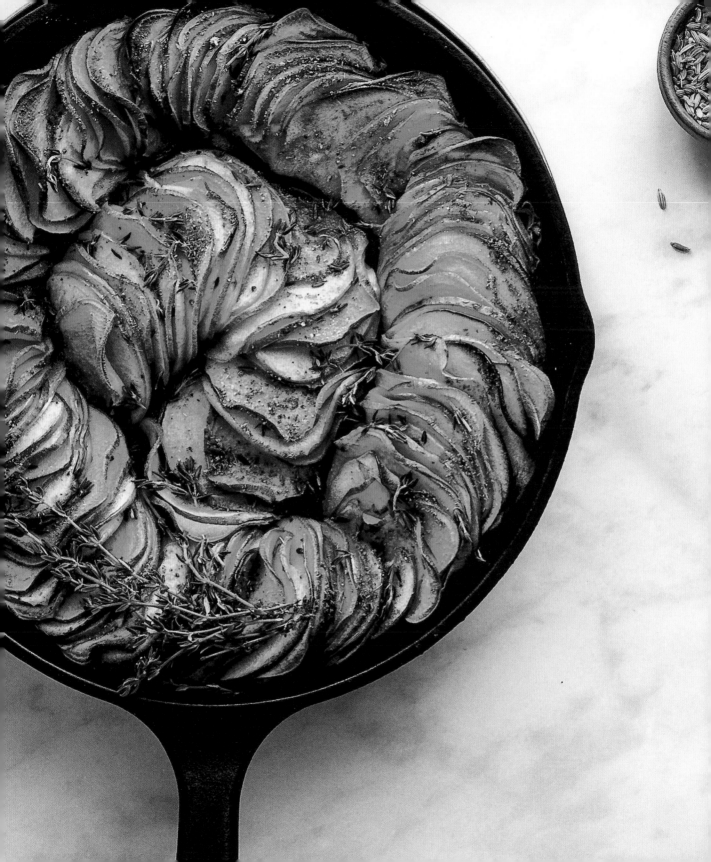

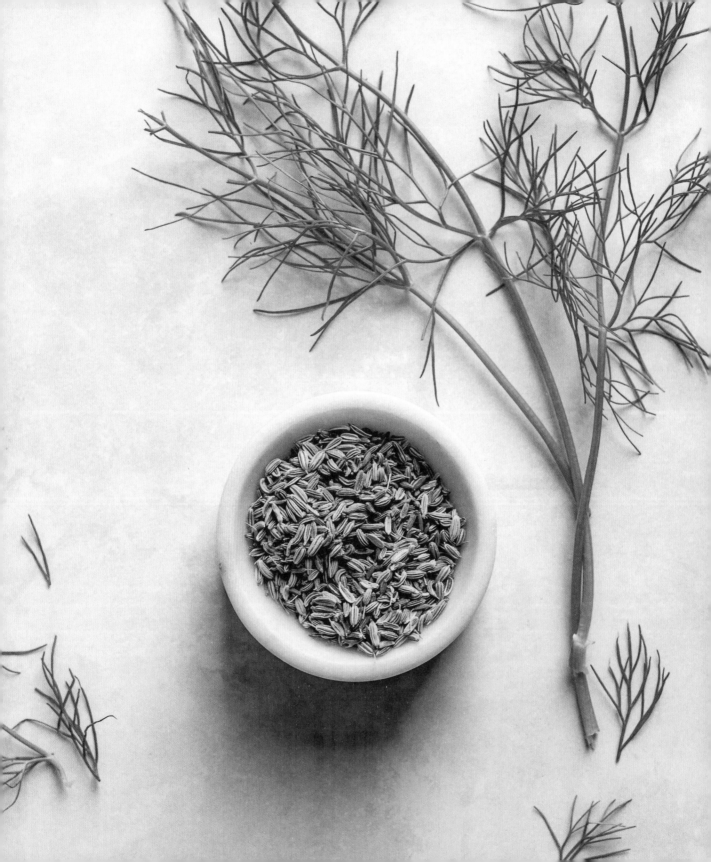

fennel
(foeniculum vulgare)

Fennel is an aromatic herb with a licorice-like flavor that's native to the Mediterranean. Its hollow stems shoot up about 3 feet from layered white bulbs that barely peek above the soil before giving way to feathery green leaves. In late summer, the tiniest flowers, each dusty with pollen, open like a constellation of vivid yellow starbursts. Later, as hot weather turns cold, the stems dry and the flowers turn to seed.

While the whole fennel plant, from its succulent bulb to the specks of pollen on each flower, is edible, the herb's seeds hold the most potent medicine. As a carminative herb, fennel seeds support digestion by easing bloating and gas, and they also stimulate the appetite and alleviate nausea. Fennel has a gentle, but potent medicinal effect. Traditionally, herbalists use the herb in gripe waters for colicky babies. You can experience the same wind-relieving effect by chewing on fennel seeds or sipping warm fennel infusions after meals.

Most of fennel's benefits come from the plant's volatile oils, which give it such a pronounced aroma and flavor. These same compounds also combat inflammation and support cellular health.

Fennel is in season in autumn. You can slice fennel bulb for salads, but it's also delicious braised or roasted. Fennel fronds, those feathery leaves, work well as a seasoning to give interest to your meals. You can also find the seeds both in whole and powdered form in most grocery stores and well-stocked herb shops. The fresher the seeds, the more pronounced the flavor and the higher their medicinal actions. Look for fennel seed tinged with pale green but full in its aroma.

Using it in the kitchen: Simmer fennel seeds in water with other aromatic herbs to make an easy digestive or grind them fresh and use as a powder. You can slice the fresh fennel bulb and add it to salads or braise it, and remember to save the fronds, which have pleasant licorice-like flavor.

herbed new potato salad

MAKES 6 SERVINGS

2 pounds small red potatoes, quartered

2 tablespoons fine sea salt

2 bay leaves

2 tablespoons Nettle Chive Vinegar (page 47) or white wine vinegar

¼ cup extra-virgin olive oil

1 tablespoon Dijon mustard

2 teaspoons celery seeds

½ teaspoon freshly cracked black pepper

½ teaspoon ground fennel seeds

1 small fennel bulb, cored and thinly sliced

2 tablespoons chopped fennel fronds

1 shallot, finely chopped

4 green onions, thinly sliced

¼ cup chopped fresh flat-leaf parsley

2 tablespoons chopped fresh dill

2 tablespoons chopped fresh tarragon

This new potato salad uses all three parts of the fennel plant: its seed, fronds, and bulbs. The fresh fennel gives the salad a delightful crunch, while the potatoes are cooked to a lovely tenderness. As a medicinal herb, fennel supports digestion through its aromatic qualities. It's precisely the herb's fragrant essence that comes through in this dish, partnering with parsley, dill, and tarragon. While we don't typically think of potatoes as a food that supports digestion, they contain a special type of carbohydrate called resistant starch that supports gut health. The trick is potatoes must first be cooked and then cooled, as in this potato salad, for that beneficial starch to develop.

In a large stockpot over high heat, dump the potatoes and pour in enough cold water to cover by 3 inches. Stir in the sea salt and then drop in the bay leaves. Bring to a boil and then immediately turn the heat down to medium. Simmer for about 8 minutes, until the potatoes yield easily when pierced with a fork. Pluck out the bay leaves with tongs. Drain the potatoes in a colander, reserving ¼ cup of the cooking water.

In a small bowl, whisk together the reserved cooking water, vinegar, olive oil, mustard, celery seeds, black pepper, and fennel seeds.

In a large bowl, combine the potatoes, sliced fennel, fennel fronds, shallot, green onions, parsley, dill, and tarragon. Stir in the dressing and then transfer the salad to the refrigerator to chill for at least 2 hours and preferably overnight.

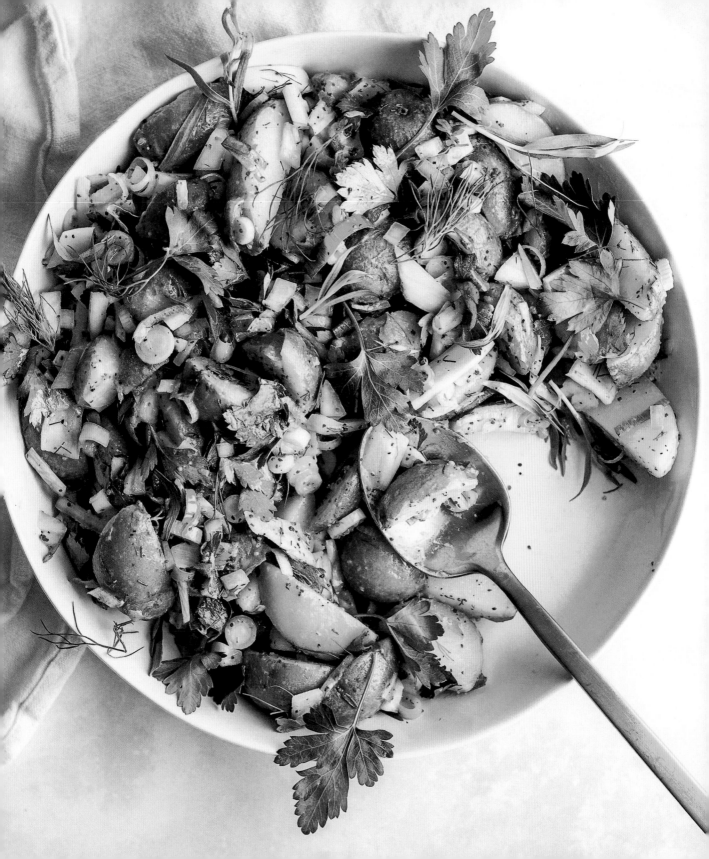

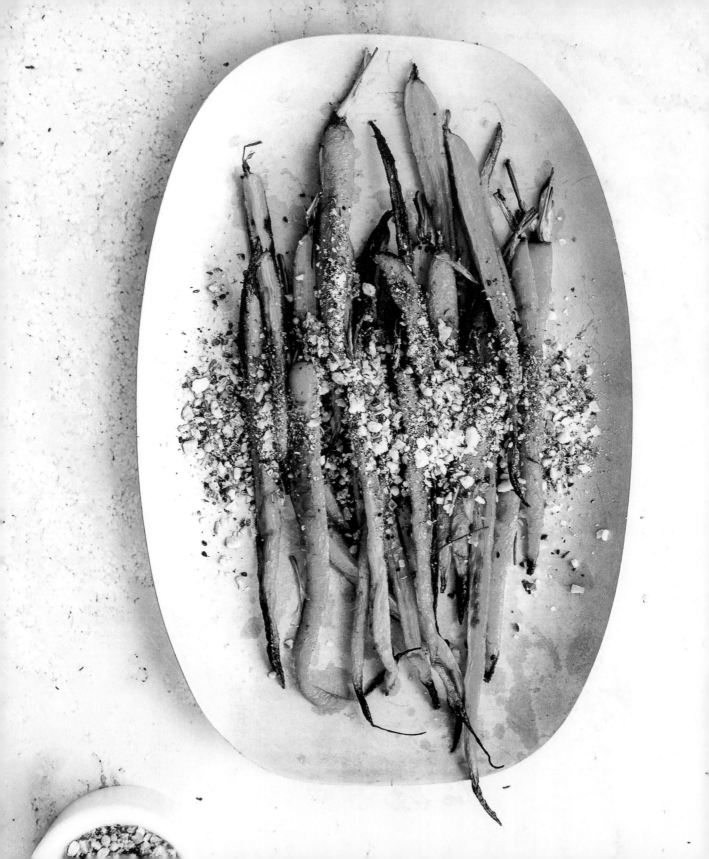

roasted carrots with dukkah

MAKES 4 SERVINGS

2½ pounds carrots

3 tablespoons extra-virgin olive oil

¼ cup coarsely chopped raw almonds

¼ cup coarsely chopped raw hazelnuts

2 tablespoons nigella seeds

1 teaspoon coriander seeds

½ teaspoon fennel seeds

½ teaspoon cumin seeds

Coarse sea salt

Roasting carrots gives them a robust, earthy sweetness and an utterly tender texture. They taste brilliant when topped by dukkah, an Egyptian condiment made from nuts, seeds, and spices. Toast the nuts and spices first and then grind them coarsely so that each bite you take gives you a flashing pop of nigella, coriander, fennel, or cumin. These bright bursts of spice bring balance to the carrot's mellow sweetness.

Preheat the oven to 425°F and line a rimmed baking sheet with parchment paper.

Scrub the carrots well and then quarter them lengthwise. Arrange them in a single layer on the prepared baking sheet. Drizzle with olive oil and then roast for 25 minutes, until their edges begin to char and they yield easily when pierced with a fork.

While the carrots roast, preheat a 10-inch cast-iron skillet over medium heat. When it's warm, toss in the almonds, hazelnuts, nigella, coriander, fennel, and cumin. Toast, stirring frequently to promote even cooking, until fragrant and beginning to color, about 3 minutes. Immediately transfer the nuts and seeds to a spice grinder or mortar and pestle and let cool for about 5 minutes before grinding them coarsely.

Arrange the carrots on serving platter. Generously scatter the dukkah over the carrots and then sprinkle with sea salt to your liking.

mint

(mentha spp.)

There are more than 600 varieties of mint worldwide, each with the characteristic cooling flavor but with subtle differences in appearance and taste. Spearmint is bright, peppermint assertive, and chocolate mint sweet. Mint gives flavor to drinks, candies, sauces, and other foods, but it's also rich in various medicinal compounds.

Once you plant mint, it'll expand out from its little patch and take over your entire garden if you're not careful. Mints have square stems and a pronounced aroma. When the heat of summer arrives, the plant flowers with a spear of tightly clustered tiny blossoms that range in color from nearly white to pale purple.

Mint is a carminative herb, and it has a strong affinity for the digestive system. Taken before a meal, it stimulates the appetite. When you sip a mint tisane, the herb relieves indigestion, bloating, and gas. Like fennel (see page 141), mint is often added to gripe waters for colicky babies because it's both gentle and effective at soothing upset stomachs.

While mint's soothing energy can ease digestive discomfort, it also relaxes the nervous system, making it a useful herb for sleepless nights, tired minds, and anxious spirits. Its cooling nature helps refresh you when you feel fatigued or overworked. A soothing mug of mint tea can help re-energize your mind without overstimulating it.

That same calm but stimulating energy can help bring harmony to other herbs, so you'll find it in many herbal blends. It combines well with ginger (see page 128) and fennel (see page 141) to boost digestion and with chamomile (see page 217) to encourage sleep.

You can find both fresh and dried mint in many grocery stores as well as herb shops. While mint tablets and capsules are also available, they contain additional ingredients such as gums, flour, and other additives and tend to be expensive, so use the fresh or dried herb when you can.

Using it in the kitchen: Add the fresh leaves to salads or finely chop them and sprinkle them over your finished dish. You can also make tisanes and infusions from both the fresh and dried herb.

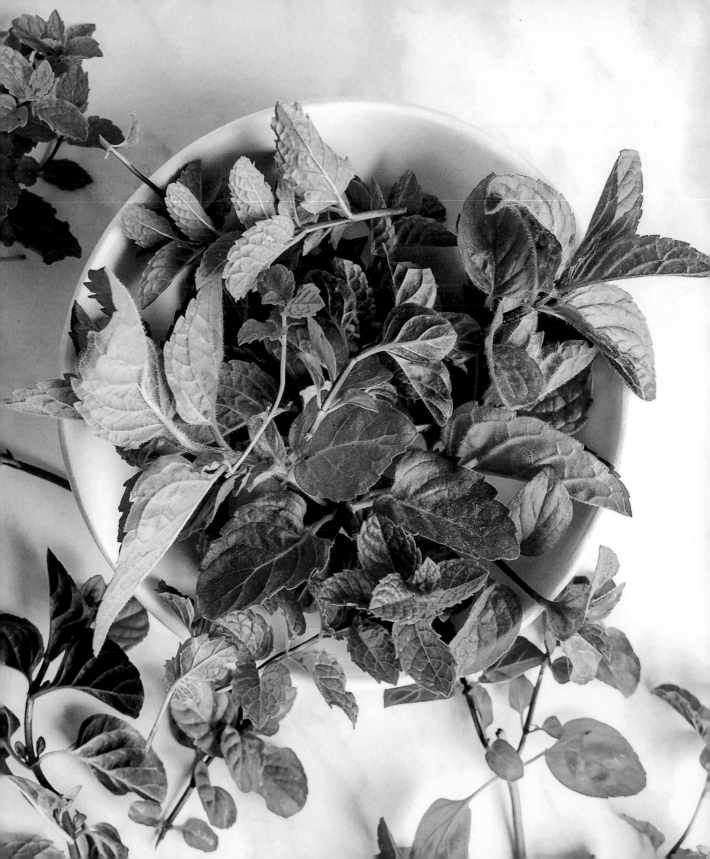

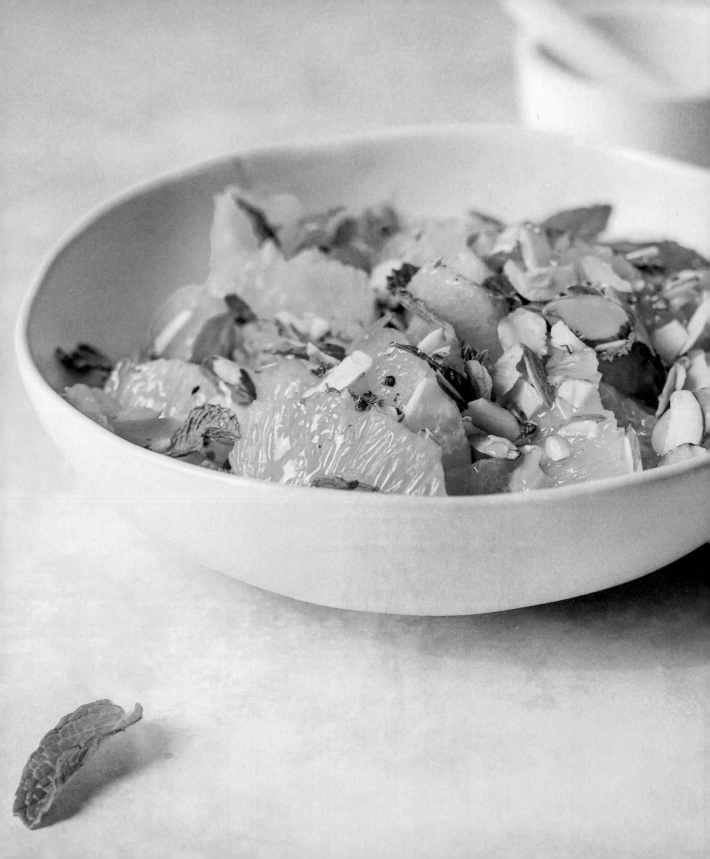

honeyed oranges with cardamom, coriander, and mint

MAKES 4 SERVINGS

4 navel oranges

½ cup fresh mint, chopped

¼ cup sliced almonds, toasted (page 81)

2 teaspoons honey

1 teaspoon orange flower water

¼ teaspoon ground cardamom

¼ teaspoon ground coriander

The vivid citrusy notes of cardamom and coriander make a beautiful match for sweet oranges in this impossibly simple, fresh dessert. Just before serving the oranges, splash them with a spoonful of orange flower water and drizzle them with honey, which brings out their naturally floral notes. Cardamom, coriander, and mint also help support digestion after meals, making this dessert not only straightforward to make but easy on your stomach, too.

Cut away the rind and white pitch of each orange. Using a paring knife, delicately cut away the flesh between the orange's segmented membranes to form supremes. Arrange the orange in a serving bowl and then sprinkle with mint and almonds.

Drizzle honey and orange flower water over the oranges, and then sprinkle them with ground coriander and cardamom. Serve right away.

carrot salad with mint and cilantro

MAKES 4 SERVINGS

3 tablespoons extra-virgin olive oil

Juice of 1 lemon

1 shallot, minced

1 teaspoon honey

½ teaspoon fine sea salt

½ teaspoon ground coriander

½ teaspoon ground cumin

¼ teaspoon ground cardamom

1 pound carrots, peeled and coarsely grated

½ cup tightly packed chopped fresh mint

½ cup tightly packed chopped fresh cilantro

¼ cup hemp hearts

¼ cup pumpkin seeds

This carrot salad is easy to make, coming together in only a few minutes. It also keeps well in the refrigerator for a few days, so you can toss the salad together on the weekend, and it's ready as an easy side dish during the week. The spices' earthy flavor grounds the carrot salad, while the fresh mint and cilantro add some brightness.

In a large salad bowl, whisk together the olive oil, lemon juice, shallot, honey, salt, coriander, cumin, and cardamom. Dump the carrots into the bowl, tossing them in the dressing until nicely coated. Gently stir in the mint, cilantro, hemp hearts, and pumpkin seeds.

Serve the salad immediately or seal it tightly and store it in the refrigerator for up to 3 days.

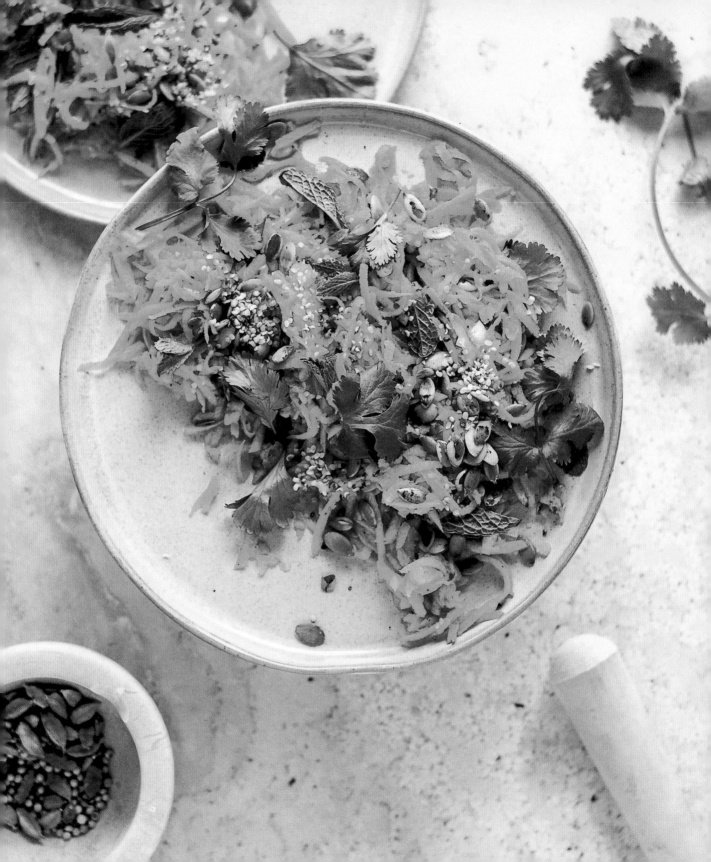

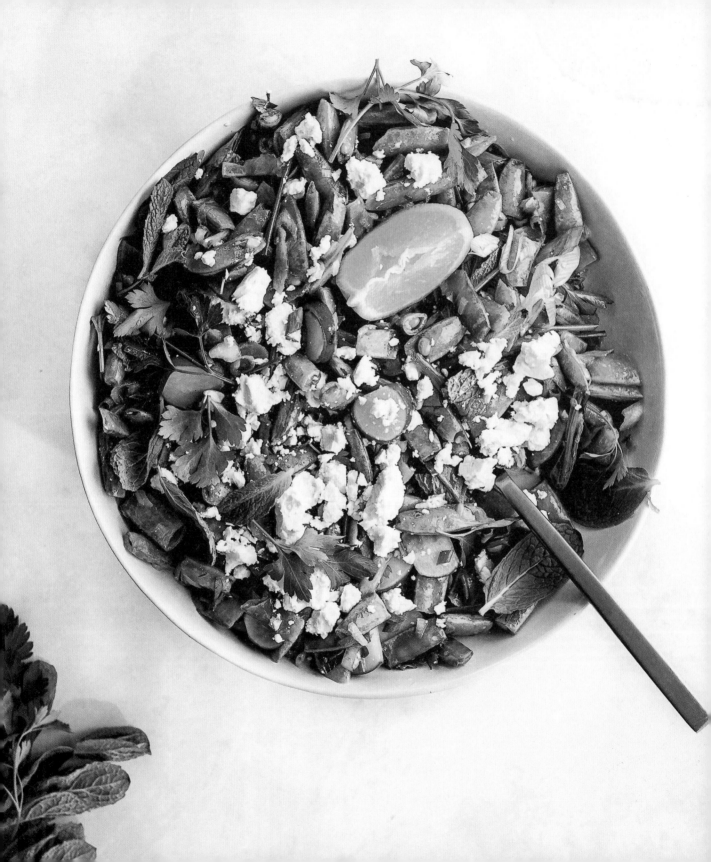

snap pea salad with mint and feta

MAKES 4 SERVINGS

1 shallot, minced

Juice of 1 lemon

3 tablespoons extra-virgin olive oil

½ teaspoon fine sea salt

1 pound sugar snap peas, trimmed and sliced into 1-inch pieces

1 bunch radishes, thinly sliced

6 green onions, thinly sliced

½ cup tightly packed chopped fresh mint

¼ cup tightly packed chopped fresh parsley

¼ cup sliced raw almonds (optional)

2 ounces crumbled feta cheese

Simple salads served in big portions are one of the best ways to make sure you're consistently getting your vegetables every day. When you add herbs to the mix, you not only enliven the flavor of the salads, but you get a boost of medicinal compounds, too. This salad is super easy to prepare because you begin by making the dressing straight in the serving bowl before tossing all the ingredients together. It will keep for a few days in the refrigerator, so you can make it ahead and enjoy it throughout the week.

In large salad bowl, whisk together the shallot, lemon juice, olive oil, and sea salt. Add the snap peas, radishes, green onions, mint, and parsley. Toss to coat everything in the dressing and sprinkle the almonds (if using) and feta over the salad.

Serve immediately or transfer it to an airtight container and store it in the refrigerator for up to 3 days.

dandelion
(taraxacum officinale)

You likely find dandelions growing in your garden every spring. Their sunny yellow blossoms spring up from milky stems and toothed leaves. In the late spring when the weather begins to warm, those yellow blossoms give way to puffy white seed heads.

The entire dandelion, from its bitter root to its softly sweet yellow blossom, is edible. The roots are rich in prebiotics, a distinct class of carbohydrates that help nourish and build the beneficial bacteria in your gut. You'll often find dandelion root in herbal substitutes for coffee and digestive bitters.

While dandelion's prebiotics, coupled with its bitter taste, make it a natural fit for supporting digestion, the herb also aids your body's detoxification pathways. It has an affinity for the liver, gallbladder, and kidneys.

Pick dandelion greens in the spring before the plants flower, when leaves are the least bitter and have a tender texture. You can pluck the flowers in the summertime to make fritters, jellies, infusions, and cordials and then harvest the roots in the fall. Always look for dandelions growing at least 50 feet away from roadways and in areas that haven't been sprayed by pesticides or other agricultural inputs. You can also purchase both dried and roasted dandelion root as well as dried dandelion greens from well-stocked herb shops, many specialty shops, and grocery stores in season.

Using it in the kitchen: Use the fresh greens to make salads, pairing them with salty and sour flavors to balance their bitterness. You can also braise the greens, dressing them with vinegar at the very end to lighten their flavor. Dandelion root makes a delicious, toasty infusion.

braised dandelion greens with white beans

MAKES 4 SERVINGS

2 tablespoons extra-virgin olive oil

4 garlic cloves, thinly sliced

½ teaspoon crushed red pepper flakes

1 pound dandelion greens, coarsely chopped

½ cup chicken bone broth or vegetable stock

2 cups cooked white beans

1 lemon, quartered

Dandelions are among the first greens to appear during springtime, and their bitterness acts like a tonic to reinvigorate the body after a long winter. Bitter dandelion greens are both detoxifying and nourishing all at once. Their forthright, assertive bitterness needs equally robust flavors to act as a counterpoint, and here we serve them with crushed red pepper, plenty of garlic, and a tart squeeze of lemon.

In a wide skillet over medium heat, warm the olive oil and then toss in the garlic and crushed red pepper. Sauté until they release their fragrance, about 2 minutes.

Toss in the dandelion greens and stir-fry for about 1 minute, then pour in the broth and beans. Simmer, uncovered, until the greens are tender, the beans warmed through, and the liquid has mostly evaporated, about 8 minutes.

Transfer to a serving dish and serve with a squeeze of lemon.

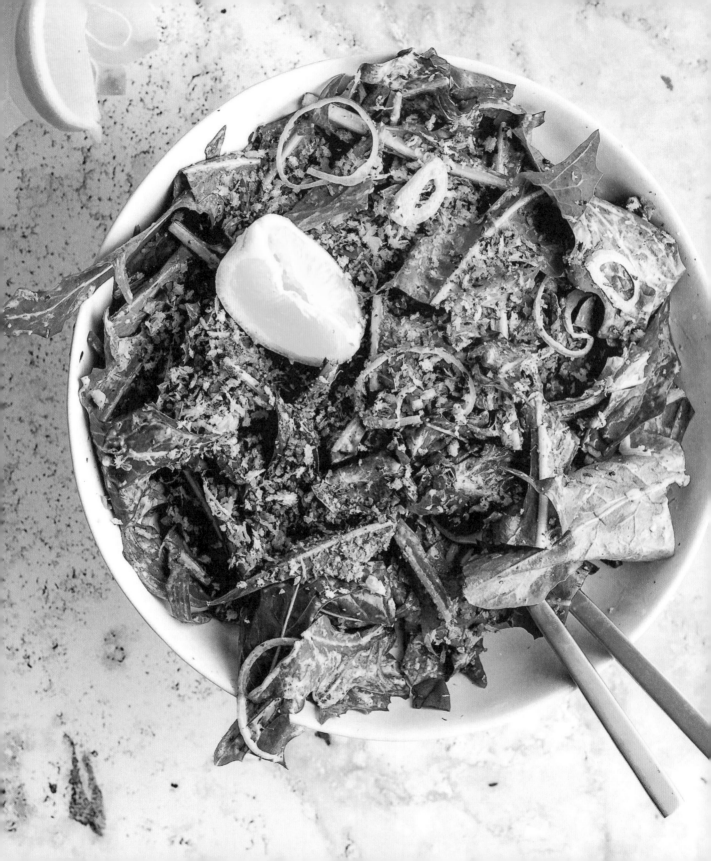

dandelion green salad with lemon-caraway bread crumbs and herb dressing

MAKES 4 SERVINGS

dressing

1 lemon

¼ cup mayonnaise

2 tablespoons plain Greek-style yogurt

2 garlic cloves, chopped

3 anchovy fillets

¼ cup snipped fresh chives

3 tablespoons chopped fresh tarragon

3 tablespoons chopped fresh parsley

bread crumbs

2 tablespoons extra-virgin olive oil

1 cup whole-grain sourdough bread crumbs

1 teaspoon caraway seeds

½ teaspoon fine sea salt

½ teaspoon freshly cracked black pepper

salad

4 ounces fresh dandelion greens, coarsely chopped

1 shallot, sliced paper-thin

Dandelion greens taste wickedly bitter, but that's also part of their appeal. That bitterness signals many of dandelion's potent medicinal compounds, the very compounds that are responsible for both its nutritive quality and its ability to support digestion.

Bitterness finds balance in salty and sour flavors, which is why the greens partner so well with robust flavors such as lemon, anchovies, and caraway seeds. The trick in using caraway seeds in this recipe is to leave them whole. Caraway powder would obscure the flavor of the bread crumbs, but when you leave the seeds whole, you'll crunch down on them as you eat the salad, allowing the seeds to release all their brightness in one bite before you move on to the next.

to make the dressing: Scrub the lemon under running water and pat it dry with a kitchen towel. Finely grate the lemon's colorful zest, avoiding the bitter pith. Set the lemon zest aside in a small bowl. Slice the lemon crosswise and squeeze its juice into a blender or food processor.

Add the mayonnaise, yogurt, garlic, anchovies, chives, tarragon, and parsley to the blender and puree to form a smooth dressing. Pour the dressing into a small jar, seal it, and place it in the refrigerator while you prepare the bread crumbs and salad.

to make the bread crumbs: Set a 10-inch skillet on the stove over medium heat. When you can feel the heat emanating from the pan, drizzle in the olive oil and then stir in the bread crumbs, caraway seeds, salt, and black pepper. Stir until the bread crumbs are pleasantly toasted, then remove the pan from the heat and stir in the reserved lemon zest.

to make the salad: In a large bowl, toss the dandelion greens with the shallot, sprinkle with toasted bread crumbs, and drizzle the greens with the dressing. Serve immediately.

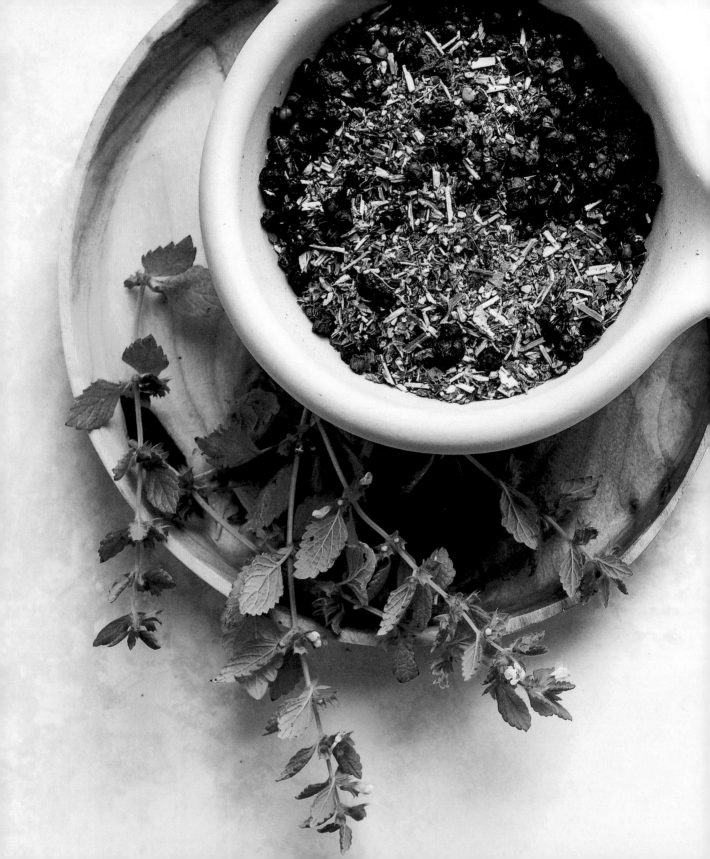

CHAPTER 6

recipes to
lift your spirit

In a world brimming with worry, it's easy to feel anxious, stressed, and burnt out. It's hard not to. While herbs don't have the power to quash the everyday stressors that can bring you down, some help build emotional resilience and support feelings of well-being. When you combine these herbs with other therapeutic lifestyle changes such as gentle movement, spending time in the sunlight, meditation, or securing social support, they can prove to be powerful allies.

If you sip lemon balm infusions over time, you might find that your anxiety lessens. When you take uplifting adaptogens such as tulsi and schisandra, you might feel better equipped to handle daily stress that might otherwise weigh you down. Herbalists have used cheerful and uplifting botanicals to lift the spirits and gladden the heart for centuries. These ancient traditions and gentle medicine provide actionable self-care that can bring solace and comfort when you feel troubled.

herbs to lift your spirit

Herbs for resilience: Adaptogens are a class of herbs that support your body's stress-response system. Herbs such as tulsi (see page 162), schisandra (see page 182), reishi (see page 104), and others help build resilience against long-term stressors that can contribute to feelings of worry or anxiousness.

Uplifting herbs: Antidepressant herbs and relaxing nervines can lift the spirit. Chamomile and similar herbs (see page 217) can ease tension and increase a sense of well-being and cheer. Many herbs in this category also work to calm the nervous system.

Herbs that calm worry: Anxiolytics, or herbs that combat anxiety, help ease worry. Some, like motherwort (see page 184), work to settle anxiousness while soothing the heart—especially good if worries make your heart race. Others, like lemon balm (see page 168), have a peaceful effect and can improve sleep, too.

tulsi

(ocimum tenuiflorum)

Tulsi is an aromatic plant with oblong, veined green leaves and small, purple flowers. The herb is native to the Indian subcontinent, and it plays an essential role in Indian culture, spirituality, and Ayurvedic medicine. It's referred to, alternatively, as "the queen of herbs," "the incomparable one," and "mother medicine."

Tulsi's diverse uses make it a powerful ally in the herb cabinet and, undoubtedly, contribute to its reputation as a healing herb of incomparable quality. In folk medicine, drinking tisanes made from tulsi daily promises to increase longevity, promote systemic wellness, build resilience against stress, and settle the mood.

By working to support your body's stress response system, tulsi nourishes you in times of stress, whether acute or chronic. It placates anxious worry. If your body is under strain due to illness, the herb helps modulate the immune system.

Like many herbs, tulsi is rich in antioxidants and anti-inflammatory compounds that give the plant the bulk of its medicinal value. These compounds calm inflammation and support cellular health by counteracting the effects of free radicals that can damage the cells in your body. Further, tulsi has a protective effect on the liver, and the herb supports and encourages your body's natural detoxification pathways.

Tulsi's anti-inflammatory properties also make it valuable in regulating blood sugar balance and supporting metabolic health. Some studies show that the herb also protects kidneys and liver against damage caused by high blood sugar.

There are three varieties of tulsi: Rama, Vana, and Krishna. Well-stocked herb shops carry all three varieties, typically in their dried form, and they work similarly to one another with minor differences in flavor and intensity. Of the three, Krishna, which has darker-colored leaves, tends to have the most beneficial compounds and the highest antioxidant activity. Accordingly, it has the most potent effect, too. When choosing a variety, try to smell each one, taking in its aroma and its energy, and then select whichever resonates with you the most.

Tulsi can be eaten fresh if you have the mind to grow it, but mostly you'll find it packaged as a cut and sifted dried herb. It makes excellent tisanes and tinctures.

Using it in the kitchen: Use dried tulsi as an infusion. If you're lucky enough to find the fresh herb, you can use it in place of basil or mint.

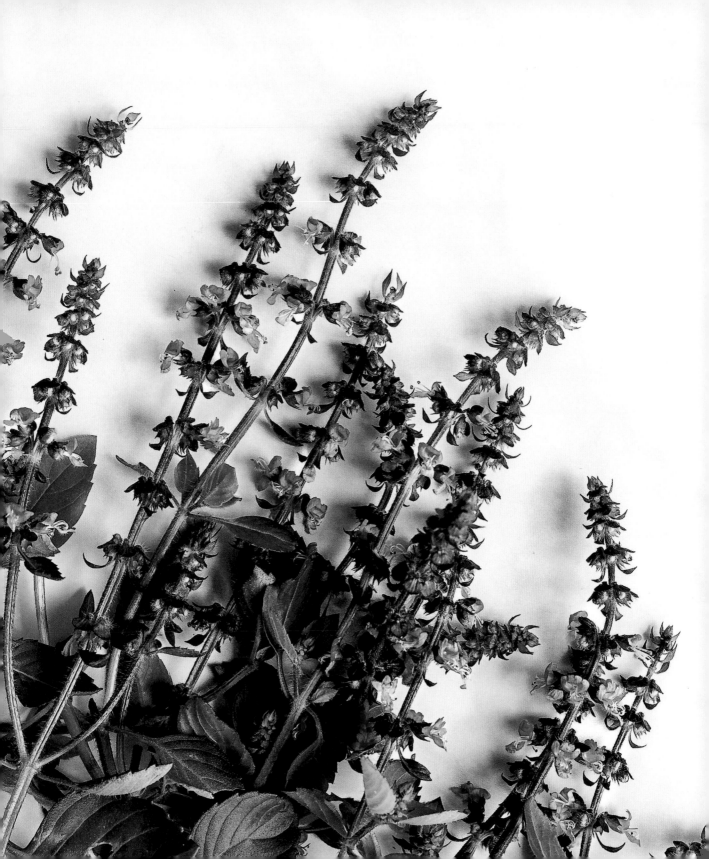

cinnamon tulsi chocolate pops

MAKES ABOUT 10 POPSICLES

3 tablespoons cut and sifted dried tulsi

1 cinnamon stick

3 cups low-fat coconut milk

1 tablespoon arrowroot powder

2 tablespoons water

½ cup Dutch-processed cocoa powder

½ cup dark maple syrup

¼ teaspoon fine sea salt

These dark chocolate popsicles are a fantastic treat. Tulsi, with its bittersweet flavor, complements chocolate well while cinnamon amplifies the herb's dusky undertones. You begin first by infusing the coconut milk with tulsi and a cinnamon stick before straining it and swirling it all together with cocoa powder and just the right hit of maple syrup for sweetness.

In a medium saucepan over medium-high heat, drop the tulsi and cinnamon stick and pour in the coconut milk. Heat until bubbles begin to appear at the edges and then turn down the heat to low. Cover and simmer for about 10 minutes.

Strain the herbs through a fine-mesh sieve into a clean saucepan, discarding the solids.

In a small bowl, whisk the arrowroot powder with water to form a slurry.

Return the herb-infused coconut milk to the stove and stir in the cocoa powder, arrowroot slurry, maple syrup, and salt. Whisking constantly over medium-high heat, simmer for about 2 minutes.

Turn off the heat and then strain the mixture through a fine-mesh sieve to remove any clumps before pouring it into popsicle molds, leaving about ¼ inch of headspace. Drop in the popsicle sticks and freeze for at least 8 hours.

When you're ready to serve, dip the molds briefly into hot water to release the popsicles. Serve them immediately, or wrap the popsicles well and then return them to the freezer where they can be stored up to 3 months.

tulsi and lemon balm lunar infusion

MAKES ABOUT 4 SERVINGS

2 tablespoons dried tulsi

2 tablespoons dried lemon balm

1 tablespoon dried stinging nettle leaves

1 tablespoon dried chamomile flowers

6 cups cold water

Thought to harness the moon's energy, because you allow herbs to infuse at night beneath the moon, lunar infusions are an exercise in herbalism, kitchen magic, and meditative intention setting. Whether you want a better night's sleep or relief from daily worries, set your intention as you pack the jar with dried herbs. Leaves and flowers work well for moon teas; their delicate nature lends itself well to slow and gentle infusions. Stinging nettle is a nourishing herb that provides a solid foundation for many herbal blends. Tulsi helps your body adapt to stressors, while the uplifting spirit of lemon balm and chamomile calms worry.

Spoon the tulsi, lemon balm, nettles, and chamomile into a 2-quart Mason jar and then pour in the water. Seal the jar tightly and set it in the moonlight. Let the herbs steep overnight and then strain the infusion through a fine-mesh sieve into a 2-quart Mason jar, discarding the solids. Serve it right away, or store in the refrigerator for up to 3 days.

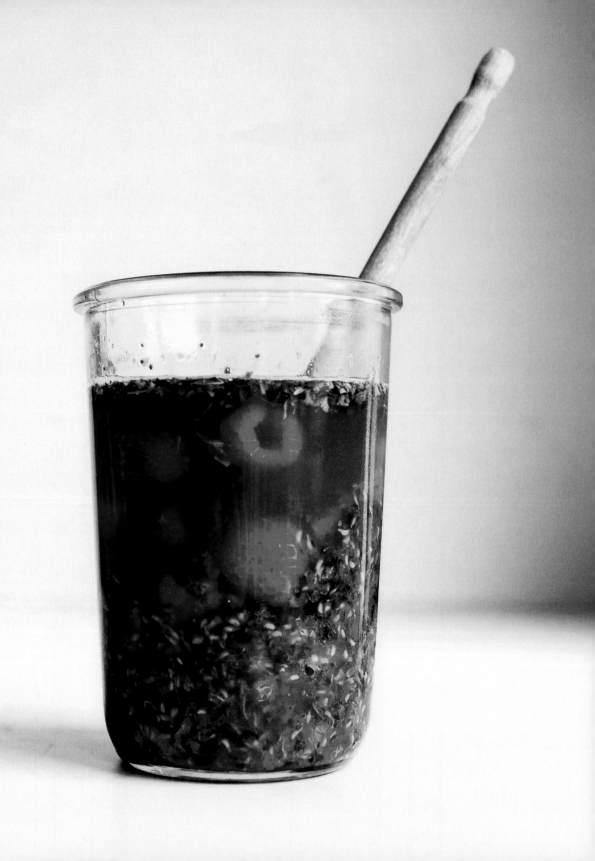

raspberry tulsi vinegar

MAKES ABOUT 1 PINT

1½ cups raspberries

2 tablespoons dried tulsi leaves

2 cups red wine vinegar

With time and minimal effort, you can make an herb-infused vinegar. Toss herbs and fruit into a jar, and then let them macerate in vinegar for about a month before straining and bottling your elixir. With time, herbs release both their flavor and benefits into the vinegar. You can use it just as you would any other vinegar: in vinaigrettes, as a finish for braised vegetables, and even mixed with honey and sparkling water for flavorful drink.

Spoon the berries and tulsi into a 1-quart Mason jar and then smash them together with a wooden spoon. When the berries lose their form and release their juice, stir in the vinegar. Seal the jar (see page 21 on how to avoid corrosion), label it, and then place it in a cupboard away from direct light and heat, shaking the jar daily for 1 month.

Strain the vinegar through a fine-mesh sieve into a bottle with a tight-fitting plastic lid, discarding the solids. Seal, label, and store the bottle in a cupboard away from direct light and heat for up to 3 months.

lemon balm
(melissa officinalis)

Lemon balm is a charming, squat plant with soft, serrated leaves and spikes of dainty purple flowers that blossom from summer to fall. It's a member of the mint family, though not as fragrant as its cousins, spearmint or peppermint (see page 146). Instead, its perfume is light, and it smells vaguely of citrus and green herbs.

Like other plants in the mint family, lemon balm has gentle and uplifting energy. It soothes a tender heart, and herbalists traditionally use it to lift the spirit. It brings light to hearts darkened with anxious worry, and it provides gentle support to an overburdened nervous system. Investigating lemon balm's traditional use, researchers have studied the herb and found it helps ease anxiety and mitigate the effects of stress, especially when taken regularly. The herb also has a slight sedative quality and promotes better sleep.

Lemon balm also supports digestive health. It is a carminative herb that helps relieve bloating and excess gas. Sipping hot infusions made from lemon balm, mint, and fennel (see page 141) is a pleasant remedy for heavy, late-night meals as it will both ease digestive upset and support restful sleep.

Lemon balm grows well in moist, rich soil away from the intense rays of the midday sun. You can also find the dried herb in most herb shops, as well as packaged for herbal tea.

Using it in the kitchen: Use the fresh herb as you would mint or basil, strewn over fruit, chopped and added to salads, or to garnish meat, fish, and vegetables. The dried herb works well in tisanes as well as long-steeped, nourishing herbal infusions.

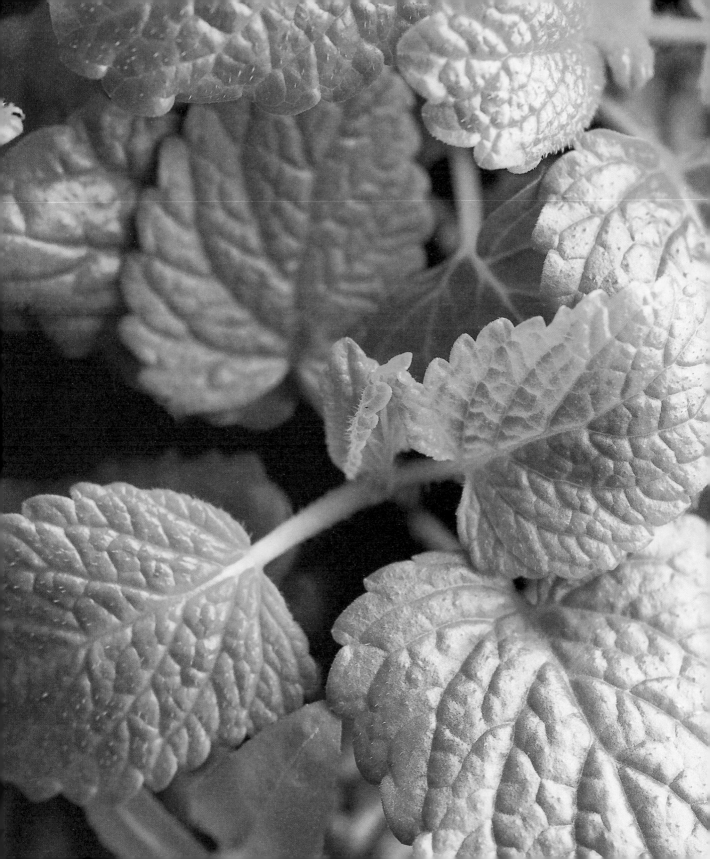

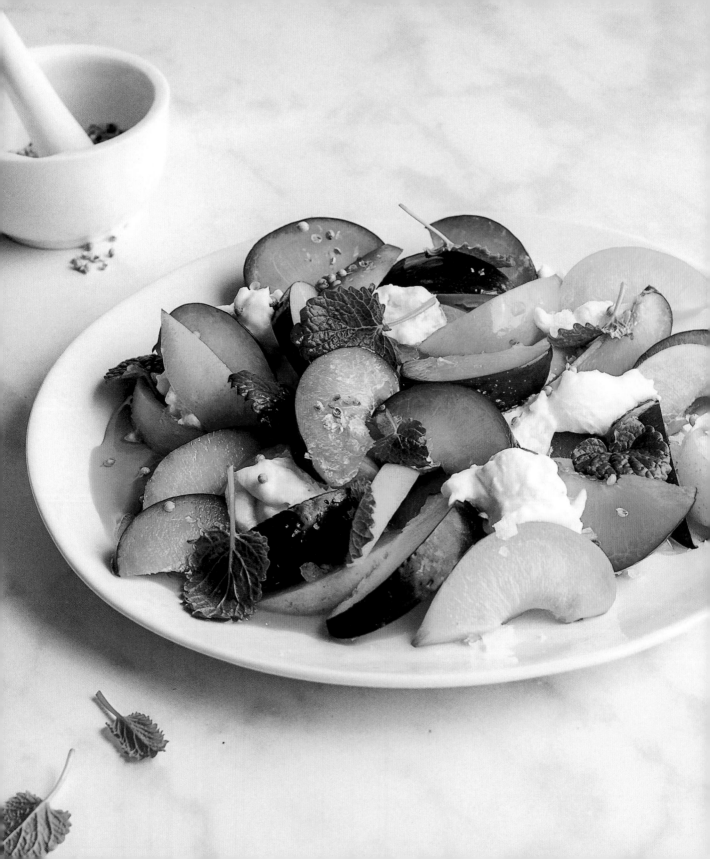

stone fruit salad with lemon balm

MAKE 4 SERVINGS

3 nectarines, pitted and cut into ¼-inch-thick slices

3 black plums, pitted and cut into ¼-inch-thick slices

6 ounces fresh mozzarella, torn

½ cup loosely packed chopped fresh lemon balm

2 tablespoons extra-virgin olive oil

1 tablespoon Raspberry Tulsi Vinegar (page 167) or balsamic vinegar

½ teaspoon coarsely ground coriander

Flaky sea salt for serving

Inspired by traditional caprese salad, we swap the tomatoes for stone fruit and slip lemon balm in as a stand-in for basil. When you toss a handful of lemon balm over nectarines, plums, and fresh, milky mozzarella in this salad, you release a sort of magic that enlivens fruit's natural sweetness. Lemon balm gives the nectarines and plums in this salad both depth and spirit. The herb's cheerful energy comes through in how it tastes, to be sure, but it also conveys that same energy to your mood, easing worry and encouraging a happy strength.

I like to serve this impossibly simple salad with a drizzle of extra-virgin olive oil and herbal vinegar, such as the Raspberry Tulsi Vinegar. If you haven't had time to make that (it takes a month), use balsamic vinegar instead because its complexity and sweetness work well with stone fruit.

Arrange the fruit and cheese on a platter and then scatter the lemon balm over them. Drizzle the salad with oil and vinegar, and then dust it with coriander powder and a generous sprinkle of flaky sea salt.

grapefruit lemon balm tonic

MAKES ABOUT 8 SERVINGS

3 cups cold water

2 teaspoons coriander seeds

One 6-inch lemongrass stalk, sliced thin

3 tablespoons dried lemon balm

Juice of 4 grapefruits

There's a sexy, mouth-puckering bitterness in grapefruit. Grapefruit's bitterness comes from a compound called naringen, which helps combat inflammation and protect your cells against damage by free radicals. Those pleasantly bitter compounds find balance in the soft, citrusy undertones of lemon balm and coriander. Together, they make a delicious, tart infusion with an earthy edge. Serve the tonic over ice on a hot summer day in place of sweet tea or lemonade.

In a small saucepan over medium-high heat, combine the water, coriander, and lemongrass bring to a boil, cover, and immediately turn the heat down to low. Simmer for about 10 minutes. Turn off the heat and then stir in the lemon balm. Let the herbs steep for about 10 minutes and then strain the infusion through a fine-mesh sieve into a 1-quart Mason jar, discarding the solids.

Squeeze the grapefruit juice into the infusion. If you're not serving the drink immediately, seal the jar tightly and put it in the refrigerator, where it will keep for about 3 days.

To serve, pour the tonic over ice and serve cold.

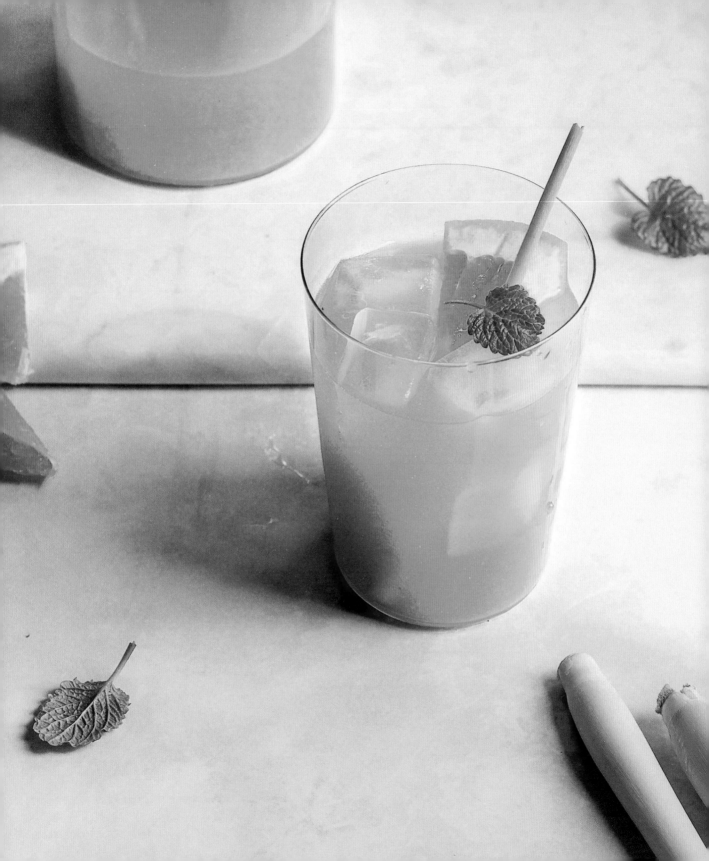

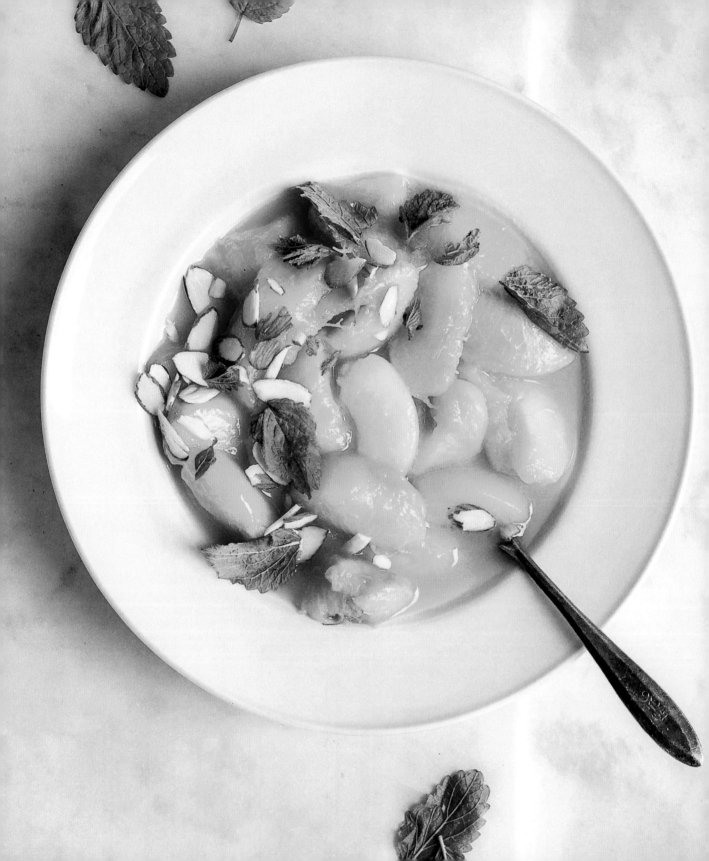

peach compote with almonds and herbs

MAKES ABOUT 1 QUART

2 tablespoons salted butter

6 peaches, peeled, pitted, and sliced ¼ inch thick

1 (4-inch) fresh lemongrass stalk, split lengthwise down the middle

¼ cup apple cider

3 tablespoons honey

¼ cup sliced almonds, toasted (page 81)

¼ cup loosely packed fresh lemon balm leaves

When peaches ripen during their brief window of late summer, make this compote. The aromatic intensity of lemongrass and lemon balm complements the peaches' acidity while balancing their sweetness. Both lemongrass and lemon balm have a gentle, uplifting quality and, when used over time, can quell anxious worry.

Regardless of their medicinal benefits, both botanicals bring a deliciously aromatic, citrusy note to this compote. Serve it on its own, over yogurt in the morning for breakfast, or with whipped cream for dessert. If you can, try to buy freestone peaches for this recipe. Unlike cling peaches, whose flesh tenaciously sticks to its pit, the flesh of freestone peaches easily separates from the pit, making pitting and slicing the fruit that much easier.

In a 10-inch skillet over medium heat, melt the butter. When it begins to froth and foam, toss in the peaches and lemongrass. Pour in the cider and honey. Let the peaches cook, stirring occasionally, until they soften and their juices form a fine syrup that's thick enough to coat the back of a spoon, about 15 minutes.

Remove the peaches from the heat and carefully pluck out the lemongrass using a fork or tongs. Spoon the peaches into a serving dish and sprinkle with almonds and lemon balm. Serve warm.

If you plan to serve the compote later, wait to add the almonds and lemon balm. Store the peaches in an airtight container in the refrigerator for up to 5 days. Serve it cold or add a couple of spoonfuls of water and warm it in a skillet for a few minutes. Then finish the compote by adding the almonds and lemon balm just before serving.

lemongrass
(cymbopogon citratus)

Lemongrass shoots up from the earth with a woody stem and long, sharp green leaves. Its extraordinary aroma, sweet and citrusy, makes the herb an asset in the kitchen. You'll find its distinct flavor in Southeast Asian cookery, as well as in herbal teas as a stand-in for citrus peel.

Lemongrass has a happy energy. While research on the herb is relatively scarce, it is traditionally used to ease worry and feelings of sadness. You'll often find it blended with other herbs such as lavender (see page 207) in relaxing infusions.

Herbalists use the herb to support digestion, especially a grumbling or upset stomach. Most of its benefits come from naturally occurring antioxidants and volatile oils that give the plant its flavor and resonant perfume. Like most herbs, lemongrass cools inflammation.

You can find lemongrass in most grocery stores. It's available fresh, chopped and dried, as a refrigerated paste, and frozen in blocks. Choose the fresh stems when you can, as lemongrass's volatile oils can dissipate with long-term storage. Avoid lemongrass paste and frozen lemongrass, or at the very least, look over the nutrition panel carefully, as many contain food additives.

Using it in the kitchen: Lemongrass hovers on the line between woody and delicate. Sliced very thinly, you can use it fresh, and it's good simmered in water for a tisane or used to season sauces and soups.

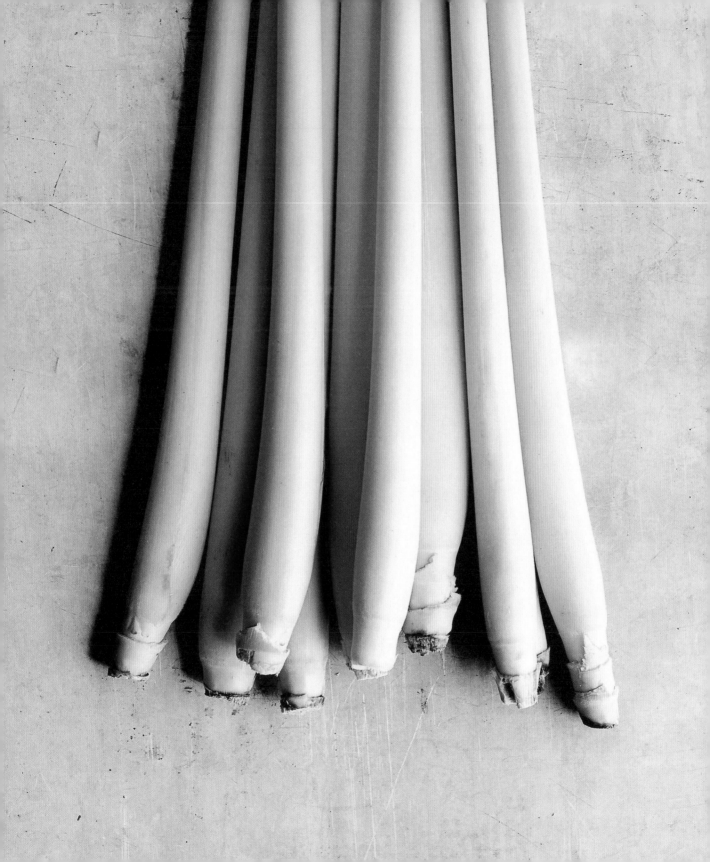

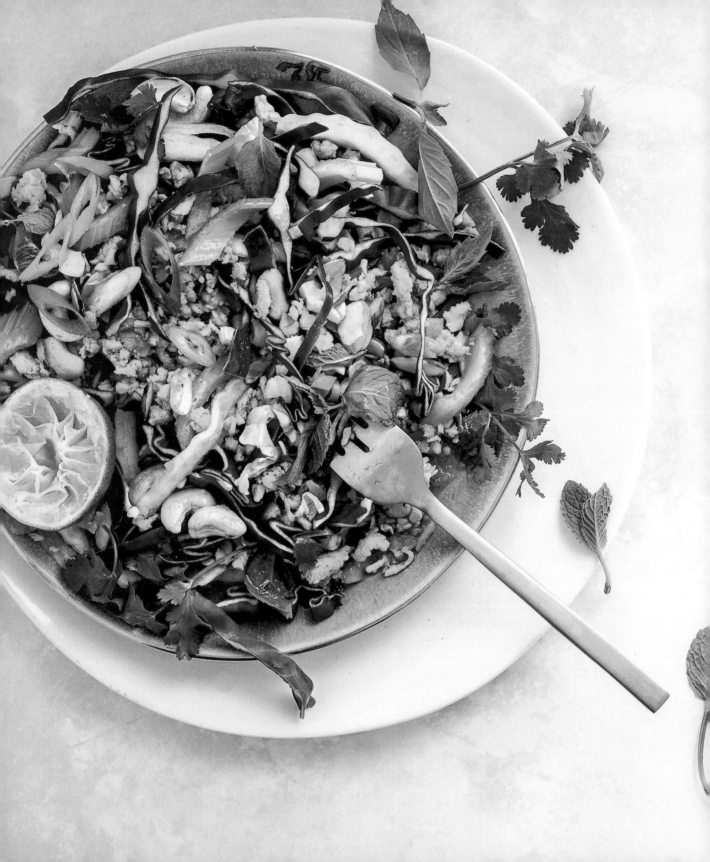

lemongrass turkey bowls with fresh herbs

MAKES 4 SERVINGS

½ cup dried, unsweetened coconut

½ cup chopped raw cashews

1 tablespoon coconut oil

1½ pounds ground turkey

1 (4-inch) lemongrass stalk, white inner part only, minced

4 garlic cloves, minced

1 (2-inch) knob ginger, finely grated

1 teaspoon ground turmeric

1 teaspoon fine sea salt

8 ounces shredded napa cabbage

8 ounces shredded red cabbage

4 celery stalks, sliced ¼ inch thick on the diagonal

6 green onions, thinly sliced

½ cup loosely packed Thai basil leaves or fresh tulsi

¼ cup loosely packed cilantro leaves

¼ cup loosely packed mint leaves

3 tablespoons sesame oil

2 teaspoons sriracha

1 teaspoon dark maple syrup

Juice of 1 lime

These bowls explode with the radiant flavors of lemongrass, ginger, turmeric, mint, basil, and cilantro. While there's a long list of ingredients, this recipe is easy to make and takes only about 25 minutes of active time.

The herbs used in this recipe have an anti-inflammatory nature, the lemongrass provides an uplifting energy, and even the turkey conveys benefits. Turkey is rich in tryptophan, an amino acid that acts as a precursor for the hormone serotonin. Among serotonin's many roles is its ability to support a sense of well-being by regulating mood and sleep cycles.

Set a 10-inch skillet over medium heat. When you can feel the warmth emanating from the pan, toss in the coconut and cashews. Toast, stirring constantly, for about 3 minutes and then transfer them to a bowl and set aside.

Return the skillet to the stove and add the coconut oil. When it melts, toss in the turkey, breaking it up with the edge of your spatula. Brown the turkey, about 6 minutes, and then stir in the lemongrass, garlic, ginger, turmeric, and salt. Continue cooking for another 2 to 3 minutes, until the turkey is cooked through.

Let the turkey cool to room temperature while you prepare the remaining ingredients.

Toss the shredded cabbages, celery, green onions, basil, cilantro, and mint together into a large mixing bowl. Spoon the turkey over the vegetables, and then sprinkle them with toasted coconut and cashews.

In a small bowl, whisk the sesame oil with sriracha, maple syrup, and lime juice, drizzle this over the salad, toss to coat, and serve immediately.

oysters with lemongrass mignonette

MAKES ABOUT 4 SERVINGS AS AN APPETIZER

1 dozen fresh oysters

Juice of 3 limes

1 small shallot, minced

2 tablespoons minced fresh lemongrass

½ teaspoon finely grated ginger

½ teaspoon coarsely ground pink peppercorns

Living by the water, we serve a lot of oysters. I love their briny flavor and the way they taste like the sea. Like most seafood, they pair beautifully with citrus, and I like to serve them with a super simple mignonette made with lime juice touched by lemongrass, ginger, and pink peppercorns.

Oysters are a powerfully dense source of concentrated nutrients, particularly vitamins D and B_{12} as well as the minerals zinc and copper. It's this dense array of micronutrients that make them a powerful ally for regulating the mood. A 2018 study analyzed scientific literature for nutrients that positively affected the mood, and its authors developed the antidepressant food index, which included foods densest in these mood-elevating compounds. Oysters were at the top of the list. Pairing them with herbs that lift the spirit makes beautiful sense and is delicious, too.

Shuck the oysters and arrange them on a platter.

In a small bowl, whisk together the lime juice, shallot, lemongrass, ginger, and peppercorns. Serve by spooning a small amount of mignonette over the oysters. Enjoy them right away.

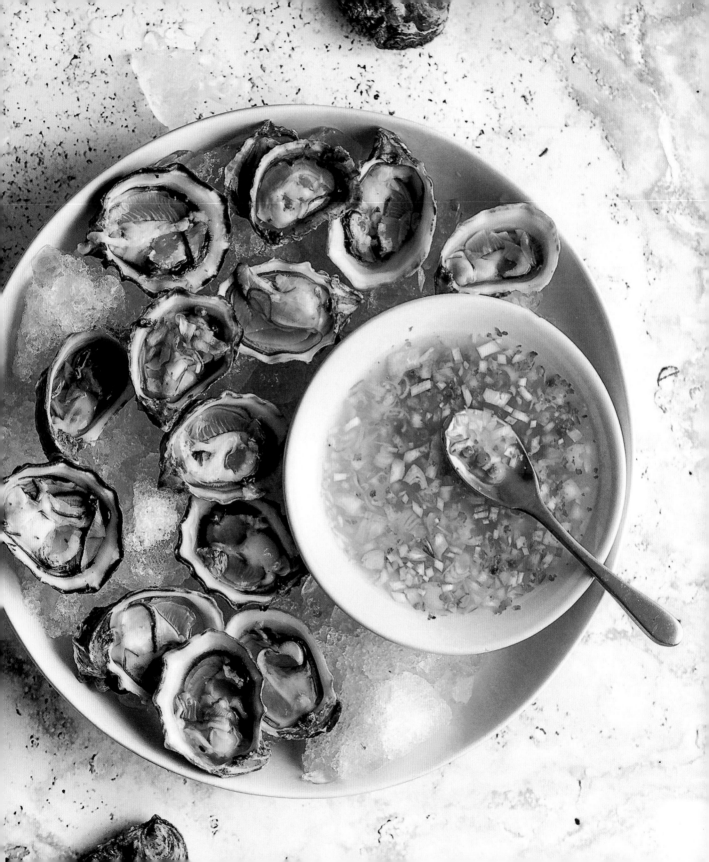

schisandra

(schisandra chinensis)

In late spring, white flowers grace schisandra vines, their centers dusted with pink and yellow. By the time autumn arrives, small red fruits hang on the vine in drooping clusters, like grapes. When fresh, the berries are a brilliant lipstick red, but drying dulls their color, making them a dark orangey maroon.

When you pop a dried schisandra berry in your mouth, you'll taste complex layers of flavor. It begins with a hint of salt that quickly fades to sour touched with bitterness. Then, as you crack its seed between your teeth, it releases a sharp, floral flavor reminiscent of black pepper. Yet, a lingering but faint sweetness underpins all those flavors. In China, where the herb has been used medicinally for thousands of years, it's known as wu wei zi, or the five-flavor berry.

Schisandra's distinctive color and potent mosaic of flavors points to the presence of several medicinal compounds. Its quercetin cools inflammation while its plentiful lignans support metabolic, hormonal, and liver health. Further, the herb contains vitamin C, vitamin A as beta-carotene, as well as trace minerals, making it both medicinal and nutritive. One of the plant's most promising compounds is schisandrin A, which relaxes the nervous system.

The herb's ability to relax the nervous system is well-known in traditional Chinese medicine, where practitioners use it to promote longevity as well as treat sleeplessness and anxiety, among other purposes. Schisandra is also an adaptogen, and it supports the adrenal glands while supporting your body's ability to respond to stress. The herb is well suited to nourish those of us who feel overwhelmed by stress and worry.

You can find dried schisandra berries as well as the powdered herb in many well-stocked herb shops. Schisandra is also available as a tincture, either on its own or compounded with other herbs.

Using it in the kitchen: Schisandra makes an excellent long-simmered decoction, and it marries well with other red berries such as currants, raspberries, and strawberries. You can also steep it in vinegar to make an herbal vinegar or the foundation for an oxymel or shrub.

strawberry shrub
with schisandra and chamomile

MAKES ABOUT 1 PINT

1½ cups chopped fresh strawberries

3 tablespoons dried schisandra berries

2 tablespoons dried chamomile flowers, or ¼ cup tightly packed fresh flowers

2 tablespoons fresh thyme leaves

1 cup apple cider vinegar

1 cup honey

Sparkling water for serving

In the late spring, strawberries are among the first fruits to come into season. They sprawl about in the garden, with their tiny red fruits nestled beneath an umbrella of serrated green leaves. You have to pick the tender fruits early in the day, or else they'll soften in your basket. Firm or just beginning to soften, they work well in this shrub because you muddle them with uplifting botanicals that complement the strawberries' deliciously cheerful spirit.

To make a shrub, you first make an infused vinegar from fruit and herbs. Later, you'll add plenty of honey for sweetness and then dilute the shrub with sparkling mineral water or swirl a little of the concentrate into kombucha or a cocktail.

Plop the strawberries, schisandra, chamomile, and thyme into a 1-quart Mason jar and smash them together with the back of a spoon until the strawberries break apart and their juices begin to flood through the herbs. Stir in the vinegar. Seal the jar (see page 21 about how to avoid corrosion), label it, and store in a cupboard away from direct light and heat, shaking it daily for 1 month.

Strain the vinegar through a fine-mesh sieve into a bottle with a tight-fitting plastic lid, discarding the solids. Stir the honey into the vinegar, cap the bottle, and store in the cupboard away from direct light and heat for up to 3 months or in the refrigerator for up to 6 months.

To serve, fill a glass with ice and then measure 2 tablespoons of the shrub over the ice. Fill the glass with sparkling water, stir, and serve.

motherwort

(leonurus cardiaca)

Motherwort soothes an anxious heart. Its Latin name, *Leonurus cardiaca*, means lionhearted, and motherwort is an ally for both the physical heart as well as the spiritual heart—the seat of your emotions. When worry leaves your heart pounding, motherwort provides relief. Its gentle action calms your nerves while fortifying both your heart and your spirit.

The plant grows in tall spikes with long, toothed leaves that cling to a square stem. In the summertime, tiny pale purple flowers bloom where the leaves meet the stem, and then you know it's time to harvest. From the ground up, the entire plant is edible: stems, leaves, and flowers. Once dried, you can use motherwort in tinctures and herbal vinegars or, less commonly, in infusions.

While motherwort is a member of the mint family, it's not aromatic. Instead, it strikes your tongue with an arresting, mouth-puckering bitterness. Don't let that put you off, because it's a powerful healing herb. Glycosides, bitter compounds found in plants, give motherwort its characteristic flavor and beneficial effects. They show significant antioxidant, anti-inflammatory, and antitumor activity. They also help protect the liver and support metabolic health.

The name *motherwort* means "mother's herb." In European traditions, herbalists historically used the herb to lessen the afterpains of childbirth. It can ease uncomfortable menstrual cramping while soothing cyclical irritability and anxiety. The plant also holds a sacred place in supporting the transition of menopause. For these reasons, the herb traditionally held a sacred place as a woman's herb, but its gentle medicine can benefit just about anyone whose heart needs soothing.

Herbalists have used motherwort for centuries to support healthy sleep and improve anxiety. Recently, researchers from Russia, where motherwort enjoys a long tradition of use, conducted a small study into the herb's anti-anxiety effects. They found that 80 percent of subjects experienced a moderate to significant improvement in anxiety and depression when taking a motherwort extract.

Although motherwort is native to Eastern Europe and Central Asia, it grows throughout the world. Choose dried motherwort or motherwort tincture from a reputable source.

Using it in the kitchen: Motherwort's bitter flavor can be difficult to translate to everyday meals, but it works well in tinctures and bitter formulas. You can also infuse the herb in vinegar, to make a bitter-sour base for vinaigrettes.

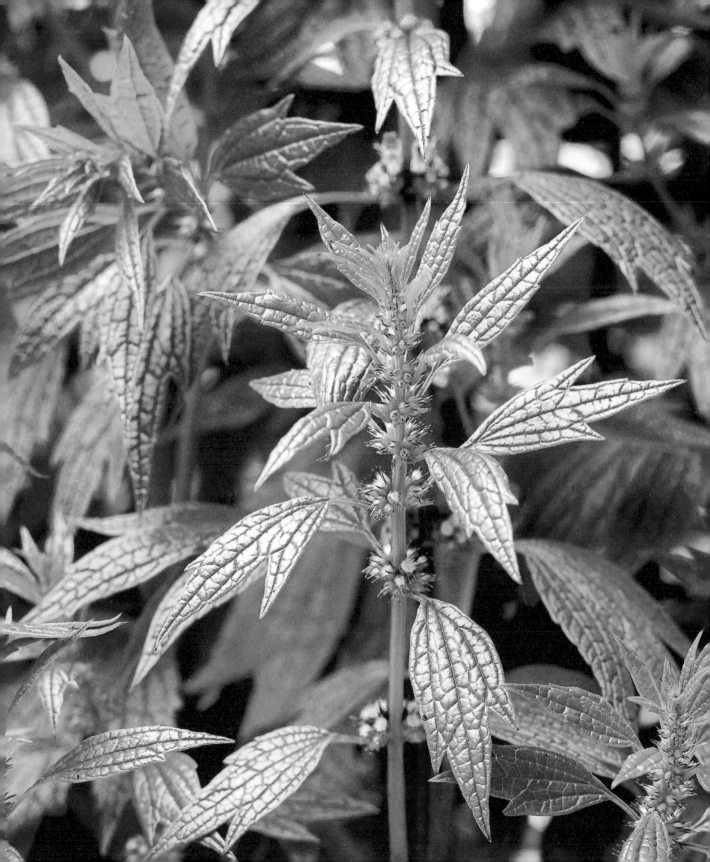

joy tisane

10 cups water

3 tablespoons cut and sifted dried tulsi

3 tablespoons cut and sifted dried spearmint

2 tablespoons cut and sifted lemon balm

2 tablespoons cut and sifted dried lemongrass

1 tablespoon cut and sifted dried motherwort

This tisane tastes minty with a subtle bitter note that comes from motherwort, an herb that lifts the heart and eases worry. It works well with other herbs, such as tulsi, which helps your body respond to stress. Lemongrass, which has a pleasant flavor and happy spirit, mellows motherwort's bitterness and lightens the tisane's flavor. If you prefer a more medicinal tonic, consider letting the herbs steep for several hours. A long steeping time, customary in traditional herbal infusions, will release more beneficial compounds but will also amplify motherwort's bitter flavor. Serve the tisane hot or chilled over ice.

In a large pot over medium-high heat, bring the water to a boil and then immediately turn off the heat. Stir in the tulsi, spearmint, lemon balm, lemongrass, and motherwort and then cover the pot. Let the herbs steep in hot water for about 5 minutes.

Strain the tisane through a fine-mesh sieve into a 2-quart jar, discarding the solids.

You can serve the tisane right away or seal, label, and store the jar in the refrigerator for up to 3 days.

motherwort tincture

MAKES ABOUT 1 CUP TINCTURE

½ cup cut and sifted dried
motherwort

8 ounces 100-proof distilled
alcohol, such as vodka

Many people find motherwort's potently bitter flavor a challenge
to their taste buds and difficult to enjoy. That's a shame, because
the herb is such a powerful ally to people who feel anxious, worried,
or overwhelmed, especially when that worry affects the heart by
increasing your pulse or leaving you with the feeling that your heart
has suddenly skipped a beat. So, if motherwort is too bitter for you
to enjoy as an infusion, try making a motherwort tincture instead. It's
often easier to place a dropperful of tincture under your tongue than
it is to sip a cup or two of motherwort infusion. You can also use it
as a bitter component of drinks, squeezing ½ teaspoon into mineral
water or cocktails.

Using a mortar and pestle or spice grinder, coarsely grind the
motherwort.

Spoon the ground motherwort into a 1-pint Mason jar and then
cover it with the alcohol. Seal the jar (see page 21 on how to avoid
corrosion), label it, and then place it in the cupboard away from
direct light and heat, shaking the jar daily for 1 month.

Place a fine-mesh sieve over a liquid measuring cup or small pitcher
and line with cheesecloth. Strain the tincture through the cheesecloth into the measuring cup or pitcher. Gather up the cloth and then
squeeze it as hard as you can to release as much of the liquid as
possible, discarding the solids.

Place a funnel into a bottle and strain the tincture through the fine-
mesh sieve into the bottle, then seal the bottle with an eyedropper or
another tight-fitting plastic lid. Keep the tincture in a dark cupboard
and use it within 2 years.

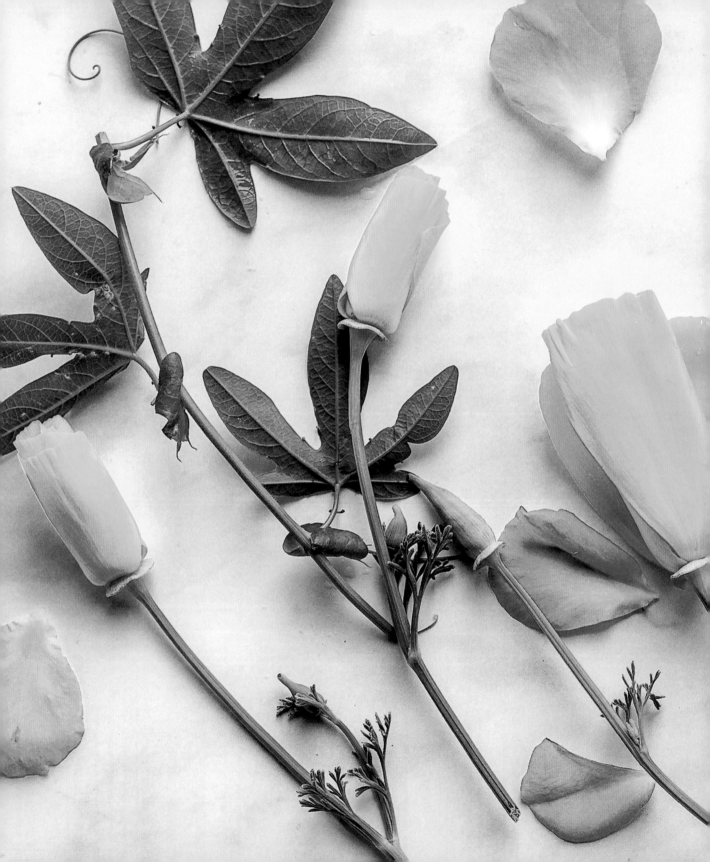

CHAPTER 7

recipes for a
good night's rest

When the sun fades over the horizon, and the sky darkens with shades of purple and deep blue, take the time to nourish yourself with mellow herbs and sleep-supportive rituals. A warm herbal infusion or a hot bath may seem insignificant, but these gentle elements of self-care provide the foundation on which you can end the day, prepare for tomorrow, and care for yourself in a way that builds and supports your body. When you sleep well and wake up refreshed and full of life, you'll have energy to tackle the day with enthusiasm and passion.

Just as some plants, such as coffee and tea, can kick-start your mornings with a boost of energy, other herbs can relax you in the evenings and help lull you to sleep. The tisanes, tinctures, and other recipes in this chapter incorporate relaxing herbs such as chamomile with sleep-promoting botanicals such as passionflower and California poppy to give you peaceful support for a good night's rest.

herbs for sleep

Relaxing herbs: Relaxing nervines, or herbs that help soothe the nervous system, are some of the first choices for those who struggle with sleeplessness. Chamomile (see page 217), lavender (see page 207), and other popular relaxation remedies settle the nerves, ease tension, and promote feelings of restfulness.

Sleepy herbs: Some herbs help support sleep more directly; these herbs include sedatives and hypnotics. Unlike pharmaceutical medications, these herbs have a gentler and mellower effect in the way they support better sleep. Passionflower (see page 202) and California poppy (see page 210) are two herbs that work well together to promote restful sleep.

Herbs that alleviate stress: Adaptogens work to increase stamina and fortify the body against stress. So, if stress contributes to your sleeplessness, as it often does, these herbs can support good sleep on a foundational level. Some adaptogens, such as licorice (see page 31) and eleuthero (see page 35), have an energizing effect so enjoy them in the morning. Others, like reishi (see page 104) and ashwagandha (see page 192), have relaxing energy and you can enjoy them in the evening, too.

ashwagandha

(withania somnifera)

Ashwagandha is a low-lying shrub with broad blue-green leaves and vivid red berries. Its natural habitat stretches from Nepal and India in the east to the Mediterranean in the west where people have used its long, woody root as both food and medicine for thousands of years.

While it's an herb of diverse and varied uses, most of these uses center around the brain and nervous system as well as the body's stress-response system. As an adaptogen, ashwagandha helps the body respond to a variety of stressors. While many adaptogens, such as licorice (see page 31) and eleuthero (see page 35), have a gentle stimulating quality, ashwagandha promotes better sleep.

Like other adaptogens, ashwagandha also supports the immune system, helping it respond to external threats without overstimulating it. You can find ashwagandha root dried and as a powder from many herb shops. It's also available in capsules, but these tend to contain additives and may be of questionable quality, so use the dried root when possible. Overharvesting may threaten wild ashwagandha, so choose organically grown instead.

Using it in the kitchen: You can add ashwagandha powder to recipes or make a decoction from its roots. It has a bitter flavor with sweet undertones, so blend it with other ingredients to improve palatability.

ashwagandha white chocolate bark with berries and rose

MAKES ABOUT 8 SERVINGS

12 ounces white chocolate, coarsely chopped

1 tablespoon ashwagandha powder

¼ teaspoon vanilla bean powder

¼ teaspoon ground cardamom

¼ cup freeze-dried strawberries, coarsely crumbled

¼ cup freeze-dried raspberries, coarsely crumbled

3 tablespoons sliced almonds

3 tablespoons dried rose petals

Vivid red berries and creamy almonds dot this white chocolate bark, making a visually stunning but casual treat to share among friends. Ashwagandha has a gentle nature and helps combat stress, while rose and vanilla bean can help put your heart at ease.

Line a baking sheet with parchment paper.

Set a double boiler atop a saucepan half full of simmering water. Dump the white chocolate into the double boiler and stir it gently until it melts completely. Stir in the ashwagandha, vanilla, and cardamom, continuing to stir until the herbs are well incorporated.

Pour the melted white chocolate into the prepared baking sheet and then sprinkle it with the berries, almonds, and dried rose petals. Transfer the chocolate to the refrigerator and let it rest until firm, about 45 minutes. Snap it into about eight pieces, or more, to your liking.

To store the bark, tuck it onto an airtight container and keep it at room temperature away from direct light and heat. While you can keep the bark for up to 1 month, it's best to enjoy it within about 10 days.

lavender ashwagandha milk

MAKES 2 SERVINGS

2 cups whole milk

1 teaspoon ashwagandha powder

1 tablespoon dried lavender buds

½ teaspoon freshly grated nutmeg

Honey for sweetening

Warm milk is a common remedy for sleeplessness, and it's all the better when blended with gentle, soothing herbs such as lavender and ashwagandha. Dairy also promotes restfulness, so skip the plant-based milks for this recipe and use whole milk if you can. Real milk is rich in calcium, a mineral with a calming and slightly sedative effect, as well as tryptophan—an amino acid that promotes calm and restful sleep.

Add just enough honey for sweetness, and for an even more relaxing quality, use a spoonful of the Vanilla Rose Petal Honey on page 198.

In a small saucepan over medium-low heat, whisk together the milk, ashwagandha, lavender, and nutmeg. Stirring constantly, heat the milk until warm and pleasant to drink, about 135°F.

Strain the milk through a fine-mesh sieve into two mugs, discarding the spent herbs. Stir in honey to your liking, and enjoy warm.

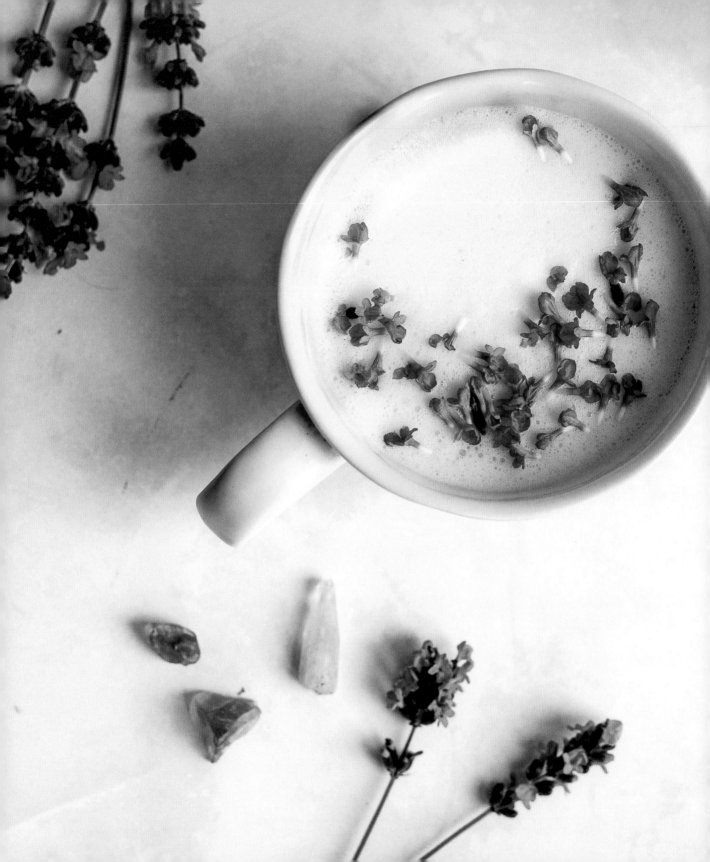

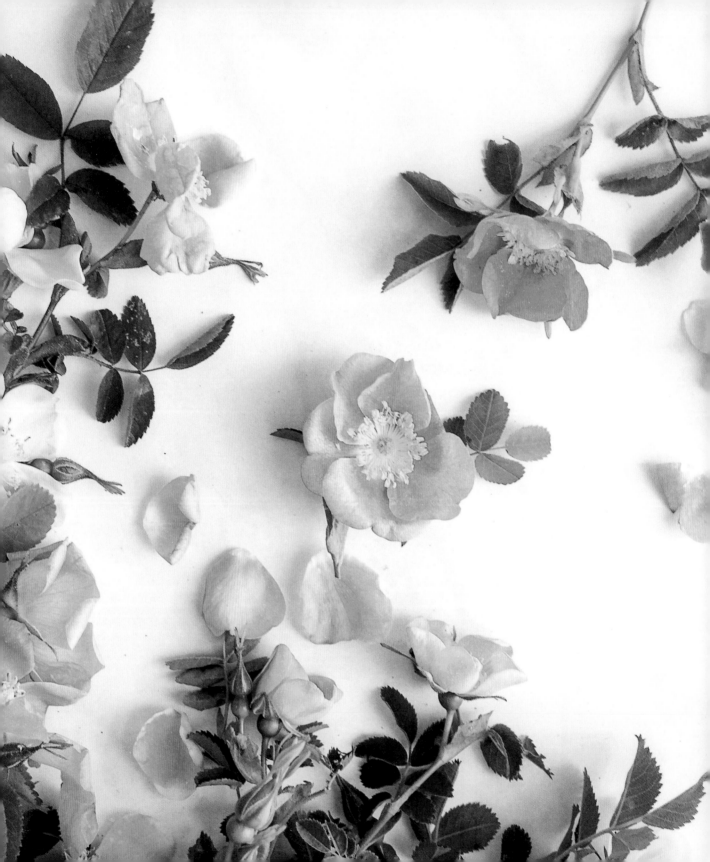

rose

(rosa spp.)

Rose, symbolic of love and joy, blooms with a burst of color and a penetrating fragrance. It grows wild in briars on hillsides and tame in gardens. Once those fragrant blossoms drop their petals, the plant sends its energy to its plump red fruit: the rosehip.

Rosehip, or the fruit of the rose plant, is a nutritious herb, providing vitamin C and bioflavonoids that help reduce inflammation and nourish the immune system. You'll often find rosehips steeped in infusions, made into syrups, or used in remedies to ease cold and flu.

While rosehips provide powerful nutrition and support for the immune system, the plant's petals and buds have a peaceful, cheery nature. Where rosehips provide nourishment, rose petals lift the spirit, calm the heart, and promote a sense of serenity.

You can add both rosehips and rose petals to infusions or make them into jams and jellies. Gather rose blossoms in the spring and rosehips in the fall from clean, unsprayed land away from roadsides and other sources of potential pollution. If you plan to use fresh rose petals, purchase only those marketed as edible or unsprayed. Roses grown for the floristry industry are heavily treated with toxic sprays that make them potentially unsafe to eat. Dried rose petals sold in herb shops and gourmet stores are intended for use in recipes and are safe to use when making herbal remedies.

Using it in the kitchen: Fresh rose petals make a delicious herbal honey, one with pronounced floral notes. Rose works well with milk and cream, too, so steep fresh rose in cream to make a rose-scented whipped cream. Dried roses make a delicious tisane but blend them with other herbs that can temper rose's robust flavor.

vanilla rose petal honey

1 cup tightly packed fresh unsprayed rose petals

1 vanilla bean, split

1¾ cups honey

Honey is naturally floral, which makes it a perfect partner for floral herbs. When you drop rose and vanilla into honey, they'll release their gentle and uplifting botanical qualities over time, and, after a few weeks, you'll have a deliciously aromatic honey that you can swirl into tea or use to sweeten your favorite dessert. Rose loses its astringent, bitter edge to honey's sweetness, leaving only its delicate floral flavor.

Spoon the rose petals into a 1-pint Mason jar and then scrape the vanilla seeds over the petals. Drop in the spent vanilla pod and then pour in the honey. Use a chopstick or wooden dowel to distribute the petals in the honey, making sure the honey completely covers all the other ingredients.

Tap the jar gently against your countertop to remove the air bubbles. Seal, label, and then tuck the jar into a cupboard away from direct light and heat for at least 1 month.

Strain the honey through a fine-mesh sieve into a clean 1-pint Mason jar, discarding the solids. Seal, label, and store the jar in a cupboard away from direct light and heat indefinitely.

Use the infused honey in place of regular honey, spooned into herbal infusions.

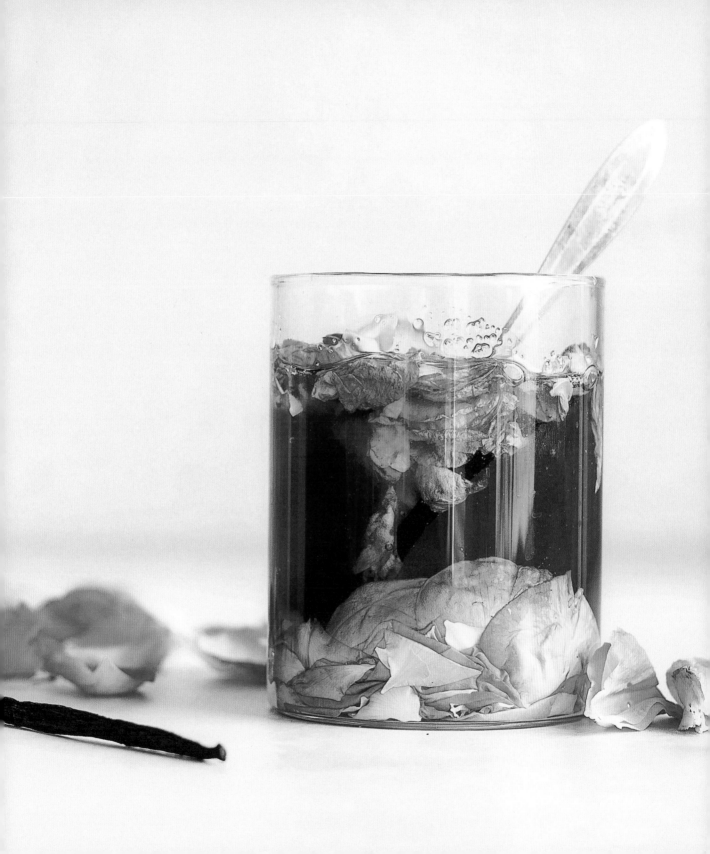

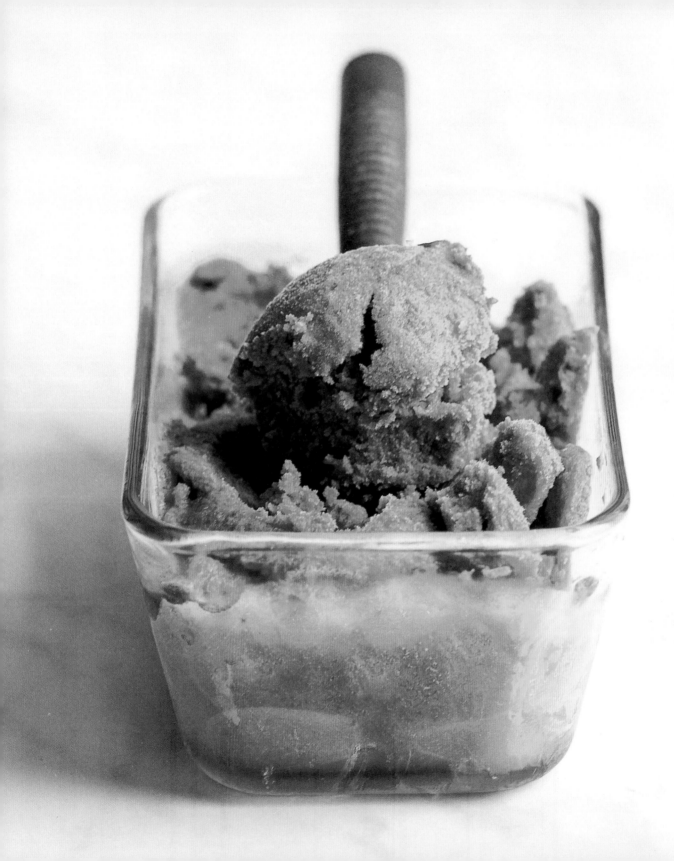

sour cherry and rose sorbet

MAKES ABOUT 1 QUART (8 SERVINGS)

3 cups pitted sour cherries

2 cups tightly packed fresh unsprayed rose petals

½ cup honey

1 cup sour cherry juice

2 tablespoons kirsch (optional)

1 teaspoon almond extract

Sour cherries are naturally rich in melatonin, a hormone that regulates sleep, and some research links the fruit to improved sleep. Rose's tranquil and happy energy provides a foundation that amplifies the action of tart cherries for a pleasant evening dessert. I like to add a few tablespoons of kirsch, a cherry-flavored brandy, into the sorbet. Its flavor amplifies the notes of cherry while its high alcohol content produces a smoother sorbet that's easier to scoop.

In a medium saucepan over medium-high heat, bring the cherries, roses, honey, and cherry juice to a simmer. When the fruit softens, turn off the heat and let it cool for about 10 minutes. Transfer the ingredients to a blender and puree until smooth.

Strain the puree through a fine-mesh sieve into a 1-quart Mason jar, then refrigerate the jar until cold, at least 2 hours and up to 1 day.

Stir the kirsch and almond extract into the sorbet base, and then pour it into an ice cream maker. Freeze according to the manufacturer's directions. Serve right away or spoon the finished sorbet into an airtight container and store in the freezer for up to 2 weeks.

passionflower

(*passiflora incarnata*)

Passionflower grows in untamed vines with ivy-like leaves. It blooms in late summer, with otherworldly blossoms. White to purple petals open to reveal thin, royal blue filaments and thick, golden-yellow stamens. As the flowers fade away, the vine forms a fruit in their stead. It grows round and hard, and as it ripens, its color changes from a bright green to a deep maroon-purple. Like an egg, the shell of the plant is both hard and fragile at once. When you cut it open, a slurry of yellow pulp, speckled with large seeds, flows out.

The fruit tastes vibrantly sour mellowed by sweetness, and it contains a rich array of nutrients such as vitamin C, potassium, fiber, and antioxidants. While the fruit is delicious, the leaves are medicinal. Passionflower relaxes nervous tension, eases anxious worry, and supports a good night's sleep.

While research on passionflower is relatively scarce, some studies show that the herb can increase chemicals in the brain that help promote sleep and a restful state. Other studies have found that regularly drinking an infusion made from passionflower leaves can help calm anxiety.

Look for dried passionflower and use it to make herbal infusions or teas to promote a restful state. You can also find it as a tincture, often blended with hops, lavender (see page 207), or chamomile (see page 217).

Using it in the kitchen: Passionfruit is delicious, with a pronounced flavor that's sweet and sour all at once. The herb has a mild flavor, and it works well in tisanes and infusions.

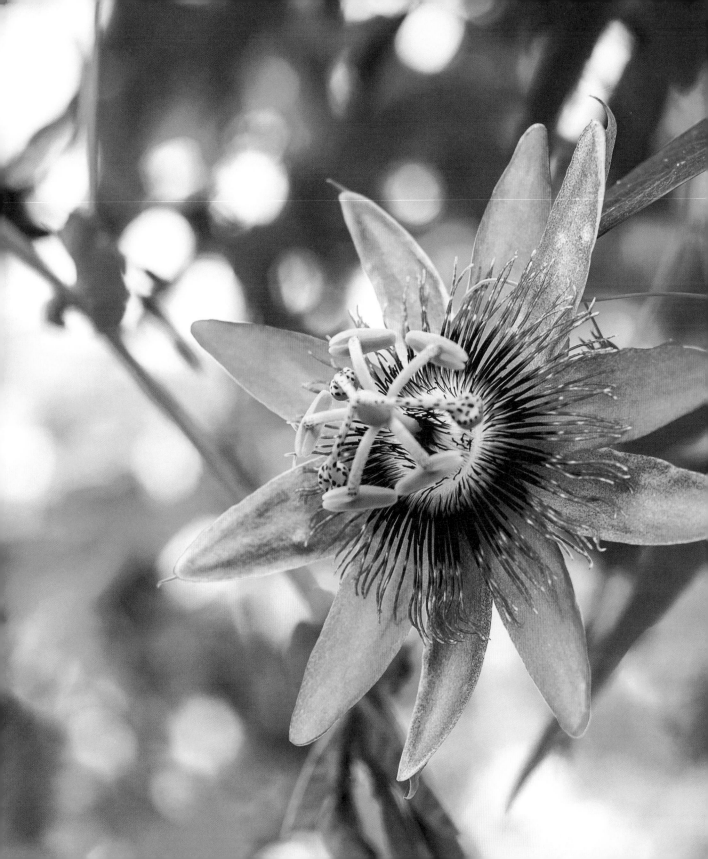

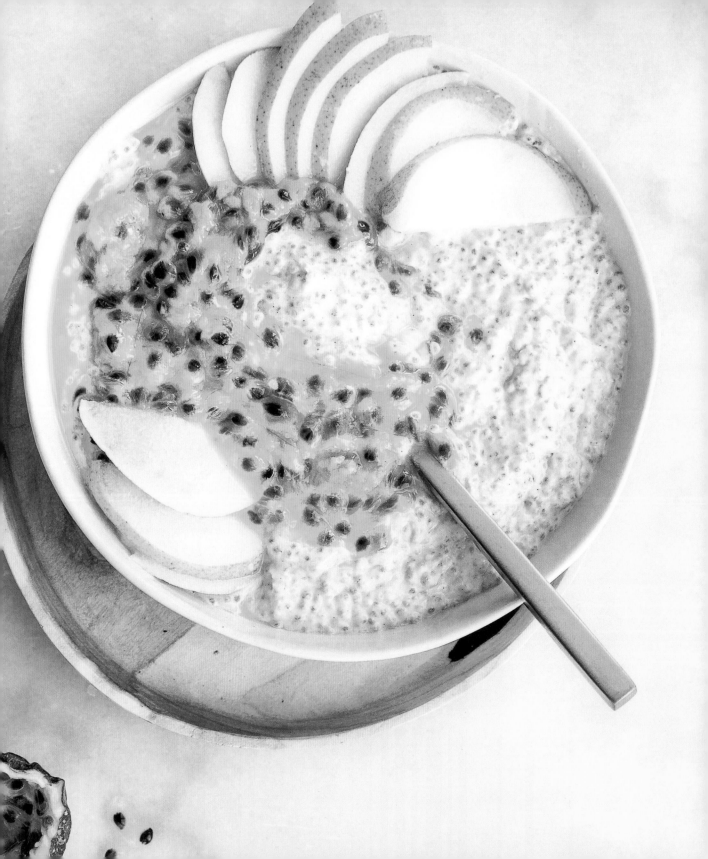

passionflower pear chia puddings

MAKES 4 SERVINGS

2 tablespoons cut and sifted dried passionflower

1½ cups boiling water

3 Bartlett pears, peeled, cored, and chopped

1 vanilla bean, split

¾ cup raw cashews

½ cup canned coconut cream

⅓ cup chia seeds

¼ teaspoon fine sea salt

½ cup passionfruit pulp (from about 4 passionfruits)

It's nice to end the day with a little something sweet, and this chia pudding is naturally sweetened with pureed pear and vanilla bean. Simmering the pears in a passionflower infusion gives the pudding a lovely mild herbal flavor, while a spoonful of passionfruit added at the end provides a touch of sweetness and punch of acidity. Both passionflower and vanilla are gentle, relaxing herbs that help lift the spirit and settle nervous tension. They're also excellent to take at the end of the day when your soul needs a little soothing.

Spoon the dried passionflower into a heatproof jar and cover it with the boiling water. Allow the herb to steep for about 20 minutes, then strain through a fine-mesh sieve into a medium saucepan, discarding the solids.

Dump the pears into the passionflower infusion, drop in the vanilla bean, and bring to a boil over high heat. Immediately turn the heat down to low and simmer until the pears soften and yield easily when pierced with a fork, about 10 minutes.

Pluck out the vanilla bean using a spoon or tongs and then transfer the pears with all their liquid into a high-speed blender. Dump in the cashews and coconut cream. Then scrape the seeds from the vanilla bean pod into the blender, discarding the spent pod. Blend until completely smooth, adding additional water if necessary.

Scrape the puréed pears into a medium mixing bowl, and then whisk in the chia seeds until no clumps remain. Let the pudding rest for about 15 minutes and then whisk again.

Spoon the pudding into four ramekins and transfer them to the refrigerator to set for at least 1 hour. Spoon 2 tablespoons of passionfruit pulp over each pudding and serve.

bedtime tisane

¾ cup cut and sifted
dried lemon balm

½ cup milky oat tops

2 tablespoons cut and
sifted dried passionflower

1 tablespoon cut and
sifted dried spearmint

1 tablespoon cut and
sifted dried tulsi

Boiling water, for making
the infusion

This soothing blend of herbs helps calm the nerves and take the edge off after a long day. It has a mellow, light flavor graced by spearmint and lemon balm. Both herbs alleviate feelings of stress. Lemon balm complements nervines such as milky oat tops and passionflower, encouraging better sleep. This blend of herbs is gentle enough for children, and you can swirl in a spoonful of honey if you like or drink it plain.

Milky oats come from the same plant that gives us oatmeal, but they're harvested young, when the plant is still green and its sap runs like milk when you squeeze the tops between your thumb and forefinger, hence the name. They're a gentle, tranquil herb that calms the spirit and supports good sleep. Find them at well-stocked herb shops (see Resources, page 226).

Scoop the herbs into a 1-quart Mason jar, seal, and then shake it vigorously to distribute the herbs. Label the jar and store it in a cupboard away from direct light and heat for up to 6 months.

In the evening, measure 2 tablespoons of the herb mix into a 1-pint Mason jar. Pour 8 to 12 ounces of boiling water over the herbs and let them steep for about 10 minutes. Strain, discarding the solids, and serve hot.

lavender

(*lavandula* spp.)

Lavender is a woody shrub with tiny silvery green leaves. In the summertime, spikes of gray-purple buds shoot up from the shrub to the sky. These fragrant buds, floral and herbal, attract bees that buzz with delight as they hop from flower to flower.

Volatile oils in the buds give the flower both its heady fragrance and its medicinal qualities. Lavender quiets an uneasy spirit, relaxes tension, and promotes restfulness. As a potent nervine, the buds can pacify nervous anxiety while encouraging a sense of peace and restfulness. The gentle way it tones and supports the nervous system makes the buds an excellent ally for people who struggle with headaches or sleeplessness—especially related to nervous worry.

Studies have found that certain medicinal compounds in lavender work within the brain to improve mood and concentration while also promoting relaxation. Further, these same compounds can reduce levels of stress hormones, too. Lavender's particularly helpful when work, stress, or travel deprive you of sleep and leave you feeling anxious or tense.

Lavender thrives in dry, sunny climates and is easy to grow. Harvest lavender just before the buds open and use them fresh or dry them. You can also buy dried lavender buds in herb shops and many well-stocked gourmet stores.

Using it in the kitchen: Use lavender buds to make infusions or grind them and add the powder to pastries and sweets. The herb is potent, and a little can flavor an entire dish, but too much will make it taste soapy.

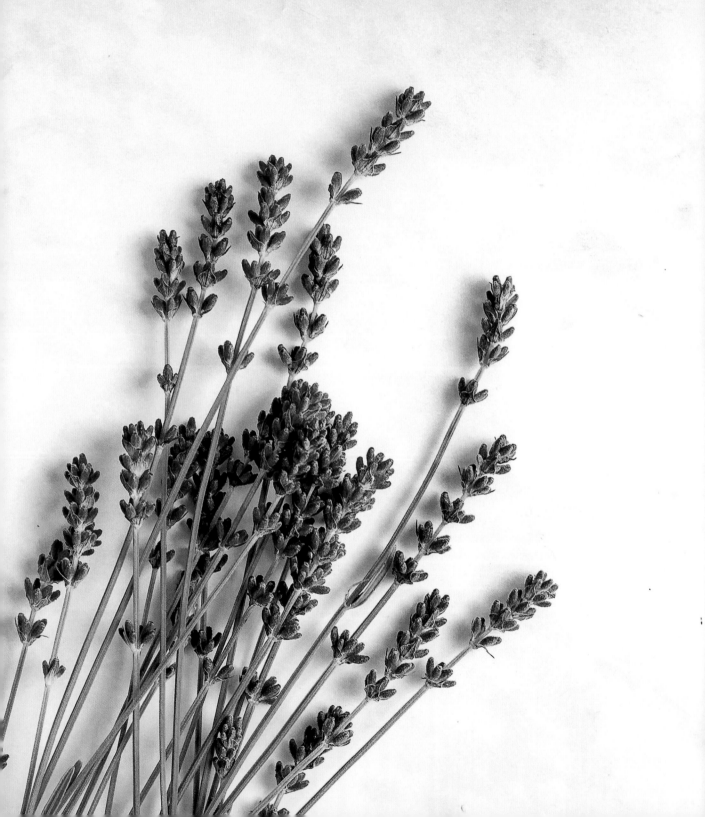

blackberry lavender tonic

1 pound blackberries

2 tablespoons fresh or
2 teaspoons dried lavender buds

Juice of 1 lemon

Sparkling water for serving

I like to serve this tonic with dinner on summer evenings. It has a pleasantly tart flavor and marvelous herbal note thanks to the addition of lavender. I serve it over ice diluted by sparkling water, but if you prefer a cocktail, try adding some gin, too. While I like the dryness of this drink, if you find that your berries are too tart, you can muddle them with a little honey to soften their acidity.

Toss the blackberries, lavender, and lemon juice in a jar. Smash them together until the blackberries release their juices.

Strain the blackberry juice through a fine-mesh sieve into a pint-sized Mason jar, discarding the solids.

Fill four glasses with ice and evenly distribute the blackberry juice among them. Fill with sparkling water and serve immediately.

california poppy
(*eschscholzia californica*)

California poppy grows wild along western North America, stretching from Mexico to parts of Canada. Its vivid orange flowers open from long stems flanked by lacy green leaves, and the herb has a happy, relaxing energy.

Indigenous peoples of the West Coast traditionally used the herb to relieve pain and aid sleep. The herb is botanically related to the opium poppy, but while both flowers have a sedative action, the California poppy is both mild and nonaddictive.

It's an especially good sleep remedy when worries, muscle tension, or stress are keeping you up.

The herb contains a wide variety of medicinal compounds; among them are various alkaloids, which give it an unpleasant and bitter flavor that you can temper by blending it with tastier herbs such as lemongrass (see page 176), mint (see page 146), or chamomile (see page 217). The alkaloids in poppy encourage relaxation and a restful state.

Look for California poppy in well-stocked herb shops either as a dried herb or in a tincture. You can add it to infusions, but its bitter flavor can taste off-putting for some people.

Using it in the kitchen: California poppy works well in tonics, infusions, and vinegars. You can also grind the herb into a powder to make herbal salts, dusts, and rubs.

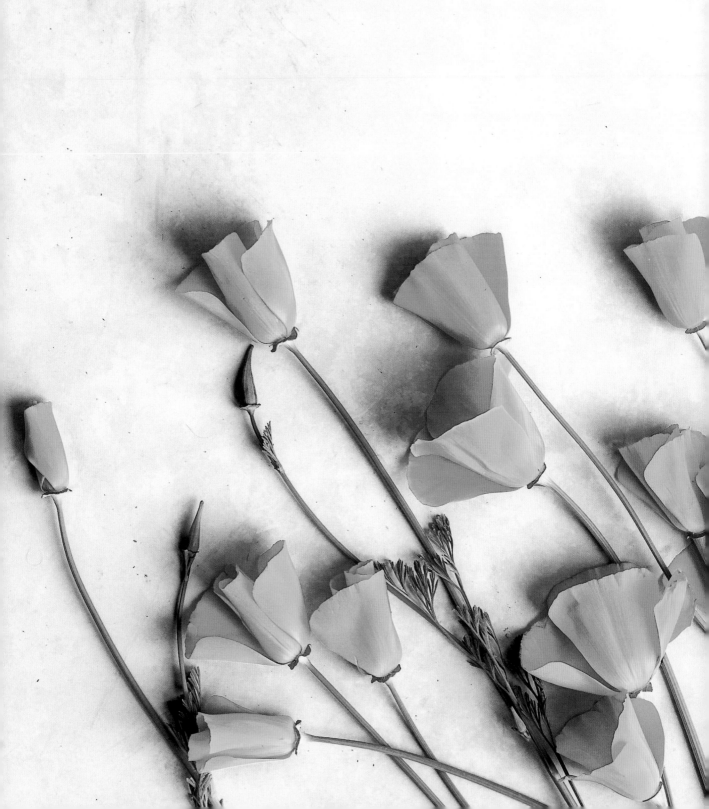

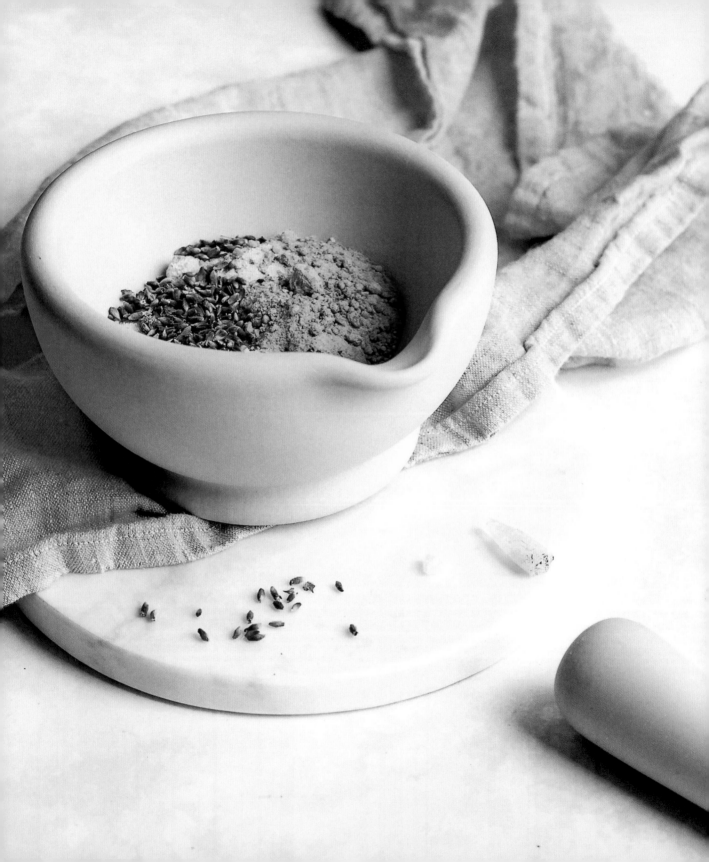

sleep dust

MAKES ABOUT ½ CUP

6 tablespoons whole, unrefined cane sugar

1 tablespoon fine sea salt

1 tablespoon cut and sifted dried California poppy

1 tablespoon cut and sifted dried passionflower

2 teaspoons cut and sifted dried lemon balm

1 teaspoon cut and sifted dried lavender buds

Salt and sugar may seem like an unlikely remedy for sleeplessness, but they work in concert to soothe the adrenal glands and promote restfulness. When stress wakes you in the middle of the night, the tiniest hit of salt and sugar can help calm your nerves, and a gentle blend of sleep-promoting herbs amplifies this effect. The trick is to grind the ingredients together into a very fine, uniform powder. If you're prone to waking in the middle of the night, tuck it by your bedside so that it's ready when you need it.

In a spice grinder or mortar and pestle, grind the sugar, salt, poppy, passionflower, lemon balm, and lavender to a fine powder.

Spoon the sleep dust into a small Mason jar. Seal, label, and store the jar in the cupboard away from direct light and heat for up to 1 year.

To take the dust, you can spoon some into an evening tisane or dissolve ½ teaspoon under your tongue before bed.

midnight flower tisane

MAKES 1½ CUPS HERBAL BLEND (ABOUT 12 SERVINGS)

½ cup dried chamomile flowers

¼ cup cut and sifted
dried California poppy

¼ cup cut and sifted dried
lemon balm

¼ cup cut and sifted dried
passionflower

2 tablespoons dried unsprayed
rose petals

1 tablespoon dried lavender buds

Boiling water, for brewing
the infusion

Chamomile and lavender calm the nerves, poppy induces sleep, and rose can lighten the heart. Blending them together gives you a light and soothing infusion that alleviates restlessness and supports sleep. As with many herbs, consistency is key, so you can make a habit of treating yourself to this relaxing blend in the evening as you ready yourself for sleep.

Spoon the chamomile, poppy, lemon balm, passionflower, rose petals, and lavender into a 1-quart Mason jar with a tight-fitting lid. Seal the jar and then shake it vigorously to distribute the herbs. Label and store it in a dark cupboard up to 1 year, away from direct light and heat.

When you're ready to brew the tisane, spoon 2 tablespoons of the herb mix into a heatproof 1-pint jar and then pour the boiling water over the herbs. Let the herbs steep for about 10 minutes. Strain the tisane through a fine-mesh sieve into a mug, discarding the solids. Enjoy immediately.

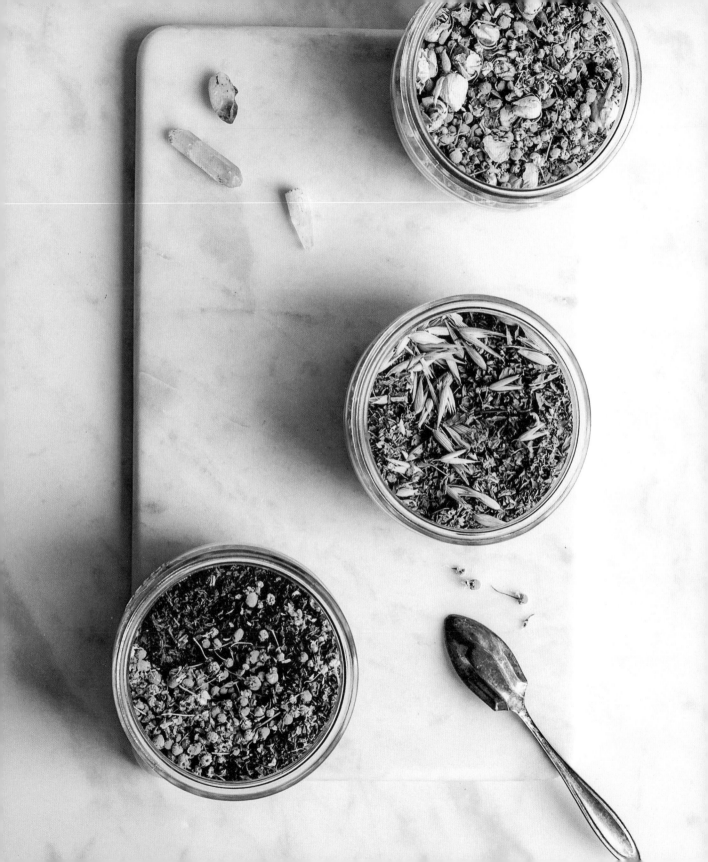

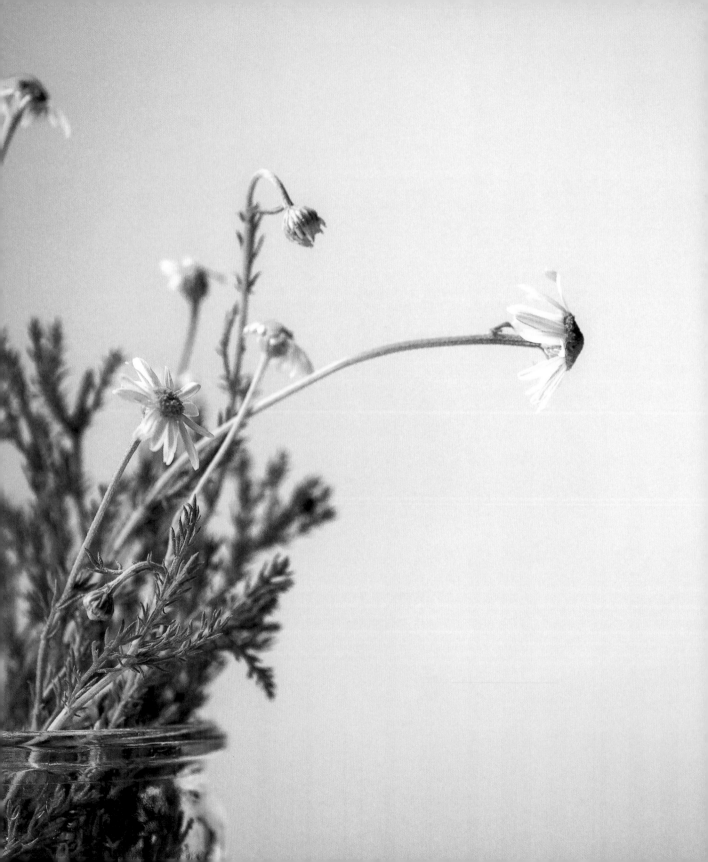

chamomile
(matricaria chamomilla)

Chamomile is an aromatic herb related to daisies. It grows with spindly stems capped by small, white-petaled flowers that droop below a large sunshine-yellow center. Beloved by bees and other pollinators, this plant releases a sweet, powdery fragrance.

With its soothing quality and gentle nature, chamomile promotes rest and tranquility, and it's been used medicinally for thousands of years.

You'll find it in many traditional remedies for sleep and rest. It lifts the mood, eases feelings of mild anxiety and worry, and promotes a sense of tranquil stillness.

The flower doesn't just soothe the nervous system; rather, it eases digestion, too. It has a mildly bitter flavor and has an affinity for the liver. It is a carminative herb used to relieve digestive discomfort, especially after heavy meals. Try blending it with mint (see page 146) and serving it after dinner for a peaceful evening tisane.

Growing chamomile is easy, whether you sow a few seeds in a patch in your garden or pots on your porch. You can also find dried chamomile flowers in most herb shops and packaged teas in many grocery stores. Look for the whole dried flowers if you can, which should be deeply aromatic. Avoid packaged herbal teas because it's difficult to discern quality. You can also find chamomile in tinctures on its own or blended with other herbs.

Using it in the kitchen: Fresh chamomile flowers are edible, and they look lovely floated in a drink or strewn over a fresh fruit salad. You can also use the dried herb to make tisanes and herbal oils and vinegars.

chamomile poached pears

MAKES 4 SERVINGS

4 cups apple cider

1 vanilla bean, split

3 tablespoons dried chamomile flowers

1 tablespoon dried lemon balm

4 medium Bosc pears

¼ cup chopped toasted almonds (page 81)

Pears ripen from the inside out, so when you buy pears at the market, gently press your fingertips against the flesh at the base of their stems. If it yields ever so slightly, the pear is ripe and perfect for poaching.

A pear's sweetness develops as it cooks, and apple cider reinforces that sweetness just enough without the need for sugar. Instead, you can build on the natural floral flavors of the pear with vanilla bean, chamomile, and the smallest touch of lemon balm. While each of these herbs infuses the pears with their delicate but pronounced flavors, they also bring a calming energy to a lovely evening dessert.

In a medium saucepan over medium-high heat, combine the cider and vanilla bean, bring to a boil, then immediately turn down the heat to medium-low. Simmer, uncovered, for about 20 minutes. Turn off the heat and then stir in the chamomile and lemon balm. Let the herbs steep until the cider cools to room temperature and then strain the liquid through a fine-mesh sieve. Pluck the vanilla bean from the sieve with tongs and scrape its seeds into the cider.

Return the infusion to the saucepan. Peel the pears one at a time, cut them in half, remove the core, and then drop them into the cider. Return the saucepan to the stove, turn the heat to medium-high, and bring the liquid to a boil. Immediately turn down the heat to medium-low, letting the pears simmer in the hot cider until they yield easily when pierced with a fork.

Arrange the pears on a serving dish, and then turn up the heat under the saucepan to high. Boil the cider until it reduces in volume by half, and then drizzle the reduction over the pears and finish by sprinkling them with toasted almonds.

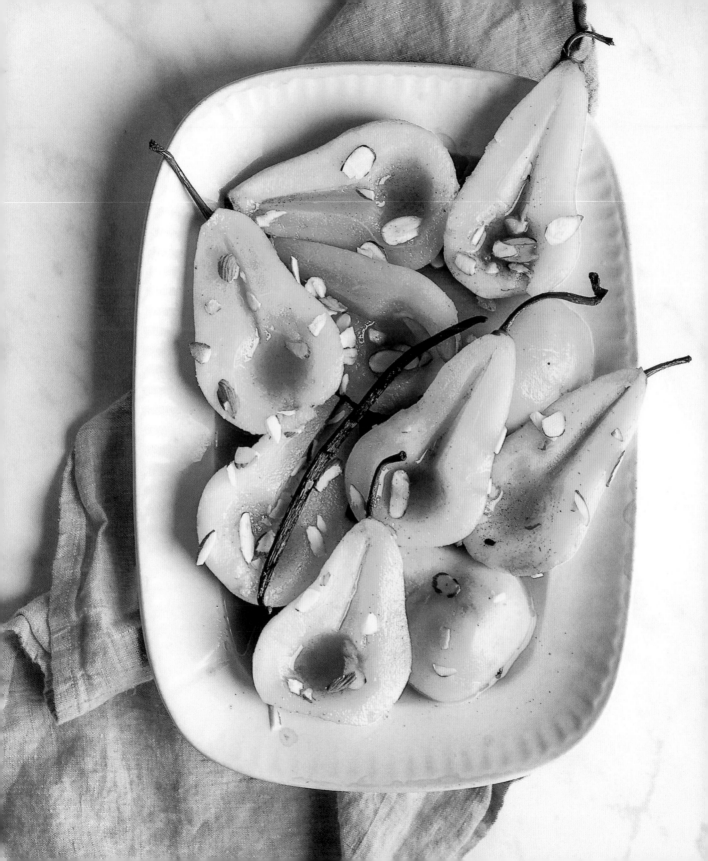

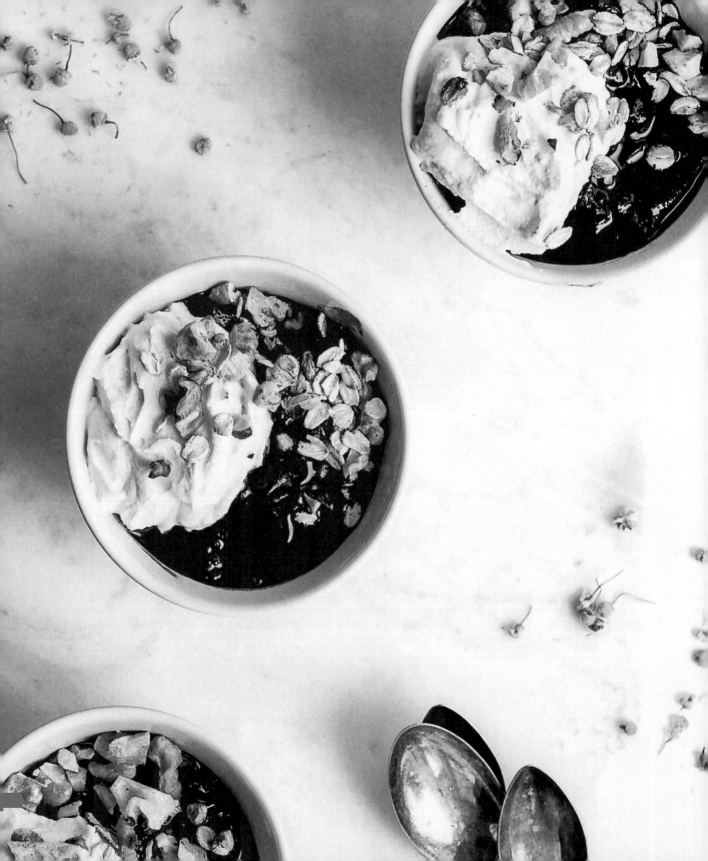

blueberry apple compote
with chamomile whipped cream

MAKES 4 SERVINGS

chamomile whipped cream

1 cup heavy cream

2 tablespoons dried
chamomile flowers

compote

2 apples, peeled, cored,
and cubed

4 cups fresh or frozen
blueberries

¼ cup unrefined whole
cane sugar

1 tablespoon brandy

1 teaspoon apple cider vinegar

oat and nut crunch

½ cup sprouted rolled oats

¼ cup chopped raw walnuts

¼ cup chopped raw hazelnuts

¼ teaspoon ground cardamom

¼ teaspoon fine sea salt

I like to top this blueberry apple compote with toasted nuts and oats for a dessert that's reminiscent of a classic crumble but decidedly less heavy. Chamomile combines beautifully with both apple and blueberries and makes an excellent whipped cream to serve with the compote.

to make the whipped cream: In a small saucepan over medium heat, warm the heavy cream. When it begins to steam, toss in the chamomile. Turn off the heat and then transfer the cream to the refrigerator. Let the cream cool for about 2 hours, until it reaches a temperature no warmer than 50°F.

Strain the cream through a fine-mesh sieve into a large bowl, discarding the solids. Whip the cream until it holds soft peaks.

to make the compote: In a medium saucepan set over medium-high heat, toss together the apples and blueberries, and then stir in the sugar, brandy, and vinegar. Bring to a boil and then immediately turn the heat down to low. Simmer, uncovered, for about 10 minutes, until the fruit softens.

while the fruit cooks, make the oat and nut crunch: In a 10-inch skillet over medium-high heat, toss in the oats, walnuts, hazelnuts, cardamom, and salt. Stir until they develop a toasty aroma and begin to brown, then transfer them to a bowl.

To serve, spoon the warm compote into bowls. Top with toasted nuts and oats and a spoonful of whipped cream.

bedtime bitters

¼ cup dried motherwort

2 tablespoons dried hops flowers

2 tablespoons chamomile flowers

2 tablespoons dried spearmint

1 cup 100-proof distilled alcohol, such as vodka

Tinctures are an excellent way to use bitter herbs whose wickedly sharp flavor can make them difficult to enjoy otherwise. These two herbs, motherwort and hops, work well together. Motherwort eases worries and lifts the heart while hops flowers promote restful sleep. The gentle spirit of chamomile provides support for these actions, while spearmint works to harmonize the blend while also contributing its own relaxing qualities.

Using a mortar and pestle or a spice grinder, coarsely grind the motherwort, hops, chamomile, and spearmint.

Spoon the herbs into a 1-pint Mason jar and then cover them with the alcohol. Seal the jar (see page 21 for how to avoid corrosion), label it, and then place it in a cupboard away from direct light and heat, shaking it daily for 1 month.

Place a fine-mesh sieve over a liquid measuring cup or small pitcher and line with cheesecloth. Strain the tincture through the cheesecloth into the measuring cup or pitcher. Gather up the cloth, and squeeze it as hard as you can to release as much of the liquid as possible, discarding the solids.

Pour the tincture through a funnel into a bottle, and then seal it with an eyedropper or another tight-fitting plastic lid. It will keep for about 2 years in a dark cupboard away from direct light and heat. Take about ½ teaspoon (2 to 3 milliliters) at bedtime.

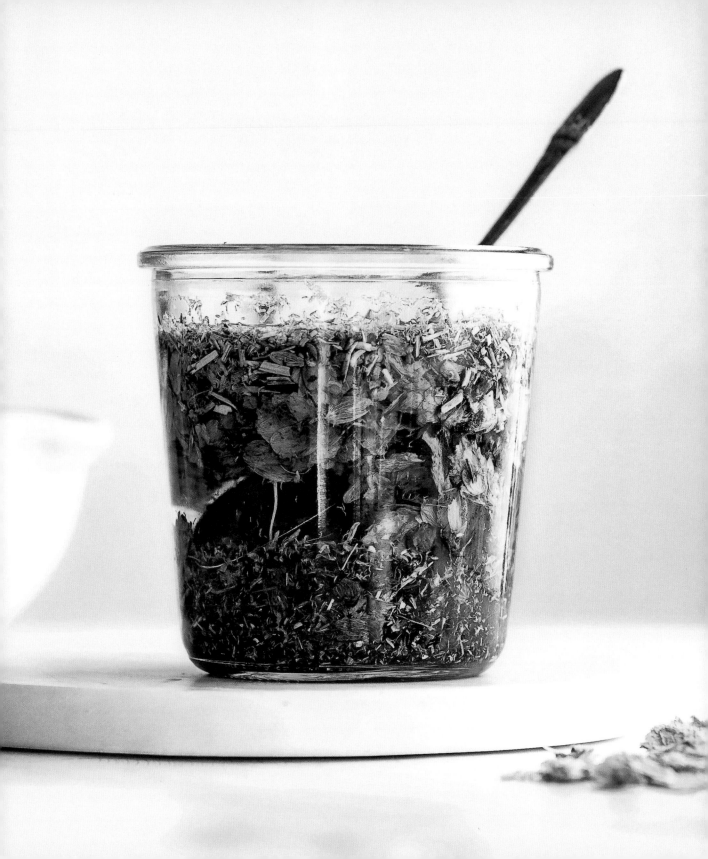

herbal safety

The herbs in this book are safe to use in culinary doses, or the amount you would typically use when you cook. Keep in mind that all herbs and spices, even traditional culinary herbs such as rosemary and thyme, contain powerful medicinal compounds, especially when you use them in very large amounts over time. Accordingly, if you plan to use herbs as part of your approach to healing, always talk with your health care provider first to develop an appropriate treatment plan. If you're pregnant, nursing, taking medication, or have a medical condition, exercise particular caution.

The table below provides general safety considerations for the herbs represented in this book. Keep in mind that even if an herb is generally considered safe, you should still discuss its use with your health care provider.

Herb	Is It Safe for Pregnancy and Trying to Conceive?	Is It Safe for Breastfeeding?	Other Considerations
Ashwagandha	No	Likely safe	High in iron, so avoid if you have hemochromatosis. May interact with thyroid medication.
Astragalus	Likely safe, but very limited data	Likely safe, but very limited data	May interact with blood thinners and medication for diabetes.
Cacao	Small amounts are likely safe, but avoid large amounts due to caffeine content.	Small amounts are likely safe, but avoid large amounts due to caffeine content.	May trigger migraines.
California Poppy	No	No	May interact with sedatives and medication for depression and anxiety.
Cardamom	Likely safe	Likely safe	Avoid if you have gallstones.
Chamomile	Likely safe	Likely safe	May interact with sedatives. Avoid if you're sensitive to plants in the daisy family.
Dandelion	Likely safe in limited amounts	Likely safe in limited amounts	May interact with blood thinners and diuretics. Avoid if you have gallbladder or kidney disease.
Elder	Likely safe in limited amounts	Likely safe in limited amounts	May interact with diuretics.
Eleuthero	Likely safe	Likely safe	Avoid if you have high blood pressure.
Fennel	No	May increase milk supply.	
Garlic	No	May cause gassiness in nursing babies.	May interact with blood thinners.

Herb	Is It Safe for Pregnancy and Trying to Conceive?	Is It Safe for Breastfeeding?	Other Considerations
Ginger	Likely safe in limited amounts	Likely safe	May interact with blood thinners and medication for diabetes. Avoid if you have gallbladder disease.
Ginkgo	No	No	May interact with blood thinners.
Hibiscus	No	Likely safe	
Lavender	Likely safe in very limited amounts	Likely safe	May interact with sedatives and medication for depression.
Lemon Balm	Likely safe	Likely safe	Exercise caution if you have thyroid disease or take thyroid medication.
Lemongrass	No	Likely safe	
Licorice	No	No	May increase blood pressure or cause electrolyte imbalances. May interact with medication.
Medicinal Mushrooms	Likely safe in limited amounts	Likely safe	Use with caution if you have autoimmune disease. Avoid if you take immunosuppressive drugs.
Mint	Likely safe	May decrease milk supply.	Avoid if you have gallstones.
Motherwort	No	Likely safe	
Passionflower	Likely safe	Likely safe	
Rhodiola	No	Likely safe	
Rose	Likely safe	Likely safe	
Rosemary	No	May decrease milk supply.	
Saffron	No	No	Avoid if you have low blood pressure or take blood thinners.
Sage	No	May decrease milk supply.	May interact with blood thinners.
Schisandra	No	Likely safe	May interact with blood thinners and sedatives.
Stinging Nettle	Likely safe	Likely safe	
Tea	Likely safe in only limited amounts due to caffeine content.	Likely safe in only limited amounts due to caffeine content.	Contains caffeine.
Thyme	No	May decrease milk supply.	
Tulsi	No	Likely safe	May interact with blood thinners and medication for diabetes.
Turmeric	No	Likely safe	May interact with blood thinners. Avoid if you have gallstones or gallbladder disease.

resources

medicinal herbs

Mountain Rose Herbs—mountainroseherbs.com
Medicinal and culinary herbs, dried mushrooms, spices, and fine sea salt.

Pacific Botanicals—pacificbotanicals.com
Fresh and dried medicinal herbs.

Pure Indian Foods—pureindianfoods.com
Ayurvedic herbs, herb-infused ghees, jaggery, and traditional Indian spices.

Starwest Botanicals—starwest-botanicals.com
Medicinal and culinary herbs.

herbal supplements

Gaia Herbs—gaiaherbs.com
Simple and compound herbal supplements and extracts.

Herb Pharm—herb-pharm.com
Tinctures and other herbal extracts.

Wise Woman Herbals—wisewomanherbals.com
Tinctures, capsules, and other herbal supplements.

healthy fats and oils

Ancient Organics—ancientorganics.com
Grass-fed ghee.

Flora Health—florahealth.com
Cold-pressed nut and seed oils.

Jovial Foods—jovialfoods.com
Organic extra-virgin olive oil made from heirloom varietals.

La Tourangelle—latourangelle.com
Cold-pressed nut and seed oils.

Navitas Organics—navitasorganics.com
Cocoa butter, cacao, and other dry goods.

Pure Indian Foods—pureindianfoods.com
Grass-fed ghee and herb-infused ghees.

live plants and seeds

Sow Exotic—sowexotic.com
Medicinal and culinary herb plants and seeds.

Strictly Medicinal Seeds—strictlymedicinalseeds.com
Medicinal and culinary herb plants and seeds.

pulses and grains

Bob's Red Mill—bobsredmill.com
Whole grains and pulses.

One Degree Organics—onedegreeorganics.com
Sprouted oats and other sprouted grains.

Rancho Gordo—ranchogordo.com
Heirloom and specialty beans.

medicinal mushrooms

Earthy Delights—earthydelights.com
Fresh, frozen, and dried wild mushrooms.

Mountain Rose Herbs—mountainroseherbs.com
Dried medicinal mushrooms.

nuts and seeds

Nuts.com—nuts.com
Nuts, seeds, some herbs, and other dried goods.

Massa Organics—massaorganics.com
Raw almonds.

sustainable seafoods

Hama Hama Oysters—hamahamaoysters.com
Sustainably produced Pacific northwest oysters.

Vital Choice—vitalchoice.com
Wild salmon and other sustainable seafood.

pasture-raised poultry

Grass Roots Cooperative—grassrootscoop.com
Pastured poultry and grass-fed meats from a cooperative of farmers.

Kol Foods—kolfoods.com
Kosher pasture-raised poultry and grass-fed meats.

natural sweeteners

Bee Raw Honey—beeraw.com
Raw, single varietal honeys.

Coomb's Family Farms—coombsfamilyfarms.com
Maple syrup and sugars.

Pure Indian Foods—pureindianfoods.com
Organic jaggery.

Wholesome Sweeteners—wholesomesweet.com
Unrefined cane sugar.

Rapunzel—rapunzel.de
Unrefined cane sugar, fair-trade chocolate.

tea and matcha

Pique Tea—piquetea.com
Ceremonial grade matcha and other tea crystals.

Mountain Rose Herbs—mountainroseherbs.com
Organic and fair-trade loose-leaf teas.

bibliography

"The Commission E Monographs," American Botanical Council, last modified 2016, cms.herbalgram.org/commissione/.

Fleming, Thomas, ed. 2000. *PDR for Herbal Medicines*. 2nd ed. North Olmstead, OH: Medical Economics Company.

Gladstar, Rosemary. 1993. *Herbal Healing for Women*. New York: Fireside.

—— 2015. *Herbal Recipes for Vibrant Health*. North Adams, MA: Storey Publishing.

Hoffman, David. 2002. *Holistic Herbal: a Safe and Practical Guide to Making and Using Herbal Remedies*. London: Thorsons.

—— 2003. *Medical Herbalism*. New York: Healing Arts Press.

Romm, Aviva Jill. 2017. *Botanical Medicine for Women's Health*. 2nd ed. Amsterdam: Elsevier.

gratitude

Writing a book is rewarding and exhausting all at once, and I am deeply grateful to the many people who helped bring this book to life. Thank you to my agent, Sally Ekus, who's been on my side for years and who worked so steadfastly well into maternity leave to help this book find its home. Thank you to Kelly Snowden for saying yes, and to Emma Rudolph for her keen attention to detail and seeing this book through. Thank you to Mikayla Butchart for her thoughtfulness and thoroughness. And to Chloe Rawlins and Lauren Rosenberg, thank you for your vision and for executing beauty in my haphazard mess. To Bella Karragiannidis, thank you for your gentle counsel and skilled advice.

To my husband, Kevin, I am so immensely grateful for you. Thank you for your care and attention and immense patience, and for always giving me the space to work. We're in it together, neck-deep and in love. Thank you for your steadfast, gentle support as I flow creative rhythms that oscillate between elation and despair, exhaustion and energy. And thank you for being such a great partner as we raise our children.

To Solas, thank you for the mountains of dishes you do. I know you don't like it, and you do it anyway. And thank you for trying everything I make, and for your love and support. To Puck, thank you for your sweetness and for learning the names of plants with me.

To Hannah, thanks for the chats and the endless support. And for listening to my frustrations (and joining me in them, too). I'm looking forward to the next time we can head to desert hot springs again. And, for my sister, Erica, thank you for always listening.

Thank you to Carol Gautschi, who gave me free reign to photograph the plants in her garden when my own decided to bloom late. To John of Spring Rain Farm, thank you for letting me peek at your greenhouse for passionflower. And thank you to Mark from Sunny Farms who scoured the West Coast to find obscure fresh herbs in the middle of a pandemic.

Lastly, thank you to the generations of herbal medicine makers who came before me. I can only hope that my work does justice to what I've learned from you and that it helps inspire the next generation's work.

index

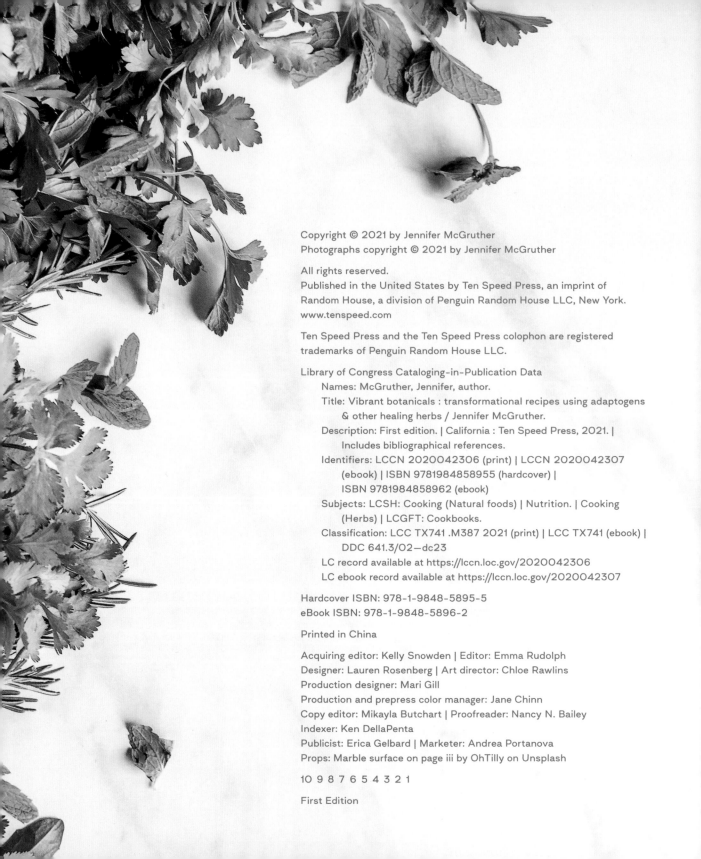

Published in the United States by Ten Speed Press, an imprint of
Random House, a division of Penguin Random House LLC, New York.
www.tenspeed.com

Ten Speed Press and the Ten Speed Press colophon are registered
trademarks of Penguin Random House LLC.

Library of Congress Cataloging-in-Publication Data
    Names: McGruther, Jennifer, author.
    Title: Vibrant botanicals : transformational recipes using adaptogens
        & other healing herbs / Jennifer McGruther.
    Description: First edition. | California : Ten Speed Press, 2021. |
        Includes bibliographical references.
    Identifiers: LCCN 2020042306 (print) | LCCN 2020042307
        (ebook) | ISBN 9781984858955 (hardcover) |
        ISBN 9781984858962 (ebook)
    Subjects: LCSH: Cooking (Natural foods) | Nutrition. | Cooking
        (Herbs) | LCGFT: Cookbooks.
    Classification: LCC TX741 .M387 2021 (print) | LCC TX741 (ebook) |
        DDC 641.3/02—dc23
    LC record available at https://lccn.loc.gov/2020042306
    LC ebook record available at https://lccn.loc.gov/2020042307

Hardcover ISBN: 978-1-9848-5895-5
eBook ISBN: 978-1-9848-5896-2

Printed in China

Acquiring editor: Kelly Snowden | Editor: Emma Rudolph
Designer: Lauren Rosenberg | Art director: Chloe Rawlins
Production designer: Mari Gill
Production and prepress color manager: Jane Chinn
Copy editor: Mikayla Butchart | Proofreader: Nancy N. Bailey
Indexer: Ken DellaPenta
Publicist: Erica Gelbard | Marketer: Andrea Portanova
Props: Marble surface on page iii by OhTilly on Unsplash

10 9 8 7 6 5 4 3 2 1

First Edition